Healthier You

Healthier You

A Family Doctor's Guide to the Fundamentals of Better Living

Vineet Nair, M.D.

ROAD

ISBN 978-0-9782077-7-9 (paperback)
ISBN 978-0-9782077-8-6 (ebook)

This book is not intended as a substitute for the medical advice of
physicians. The reader should regularly consult a physician in
matters relating to his/her health and particularly with respect to
any symptoms that may require diagnosis or medical attention.

Produced by Page Two Books
www.pagetwobooks.com

Cover design by Taysia Louie and Peter Cocking
Interior design by Peter Cocking

www.corefamilyhealth.com

For my wife, Andrea, who has always challenged
me to be better and do more than I ever thought possible,
and who continues to support me in that process.

Contents

INTRODUCTION

What Is Health?

LIVING A HEALTHIER life is the goal for many of us. Maybe you've had a health scare, watched a family member die from a preventable illness, are approaching a milestone birthday, or just want to feel better physically and mentally. But what does being "healthy" even mean? Without a clear idea of that, it's going to be very hard to know if and when you've successfully reached that goal.

Does being healthy mean looking like a Hollywood actor? A fitness model? A star athlete?

Does it mean feeling well every day, with more energy and less pain?

Or is the goal to live independently into your eighties?

We know health when we see it, but it can be hard to define. And the definition changes based on age and circumstance. When we look at a young athlete or model, we may think their physique is the epitome of health. But we often feel similarly when we see an eighty-year-old walking and smiling with no apparent evidence of disease or degeneration.

Despite our different ideas about health, my guess is that most people have the same overall goals: we would like to reduce our risk of illness, maintain our independence, and continue feeling good for as long as possible. *We do not simply want to live longer; we want to live better for longer.* Using that as our goal, it may then be easier, and more meaningful, to achieve the health status of that active eighty-year-old than that of the ripped superstar athlete.

As a family physician, I've seen patients try numerous ways to achieve their health goals, including fad diets, supplements and vitamins, unique exercise routines, meal replacements, herbal remedies, hands-on therapies (such as chiropractic therapy or acupuncture), mental health techniques, and prescription medications. While their effort is to be applauded, I often wonder if it is being applied in the right ways.

Physics has a concept of an *effective theory*, which explains what we see in the world without getting so granular that we no longer see the forest for the trees. For example, in trying to describe the action of a baseball hit by a bat (with apologies to physicists everywhere), you could note the forces of the bat, gravity, wind, wind resistance—as well as the movement of the electrons around the atoms, and then drill down even more to examine the quantum forces inside the atom—with the result that the description becomes ridiculously complex. Really, all you need to adequately describe the motion of the ball is the force and direction of the bat on it and the effects of gravity; any more granular detail only confuses the picture. It's worth applying this idea of an effective theory to how we think about health.

We are continually learning more about how the body works and what influences our health on a cellular level. However, I'm not sure this additional information is providing us with much more benefit on a practical level. The vast majority of our well-being still derives from those areas that we knew were important fifty to a hundred years ago. We should stop looking for the magic pill, supplement, activity, or device and instead consider an *effective theory of health* that can help focus our actions toward what's important: the ultimate goal of a long and healthy life.

Healthier You outlines the key areas in which to apply your hard work and energy. My intention is to break down a healthy lifestyle into actions that make an actual difference and to help you ignore all of the expensive, time-consuming, inconvenient, and sometime dangerous practices and products that don't. The focus is on improving your health by choosing from a list of behaviors that have been shown to be consistently effective. In doing so, everyone can find a number of specific ways to be healthier, as opposed to striving toward a vague definition of being healthy.

I summarize health into ten essential factors that will help guide your time and energy when trying to be well.

- Think
- Change
- Eat
- Move
- Sleep
- Enjoy
- Quit
- Vaccinate
- Screen
- Supplement?

Just imagine how your health could improve if you concentrated your efforts on making positive changes, even small ones, in these specific areas. Each chapter clarifies any confusing messages around its topic and provides specific actions to assist you on your next steps toward wellness.

While a lot of the information presented here may sound like common sense, that is the point—you already know the basics of healthy living but you need to implement them into your hectic modern life.

This book will teach you to take a "big picture" approach to health, so you can concentrate on the major areas that make the largest impact on your overall health. This comprehensive outlook to wellness is one of the main reasons I decided to become a family physician and not a specialist. My job is to be the quarterback for my patients' health and to help them navigate the complicated world of medicine. My patients receive lots of recommendations from specialists, health groups, disease-specific guidelines, celebrities, gurus, advertisements, and even other patients. It is up to me to discuss these recommendations with my patient and together decide upon the best course of action for that specific individual. I don't focus on one organ or one system but rather on one patient.

Even though each patient is unique, it is useful and comforting to know that there are basic guidelines for health that apply to everyone. That is what this book is about. While there are numerous conditions I treat and manage that require medical intervention, the ten factors described here all play a significant role regardless of your underlying health status. My hope is that this book can help doctors and patients spend our time better, individually and together, and create better health outcomes overall.

How to Use This Book

This practical manual targets key areas of health that are worthy of your focus and effort. Each section provides advice, tips, and strategies that you can implement immediately. Any references I mention are listed in the References section at the back of the book, and any useful resources and links are available at www.corefamilyheath.com/healthieryou.

You are welcome to read the chapters in any order you wish, depending on your interest and area of concern. I would recommend you work on specific areas individually rather than trying to make too many changes at once. There is a rationale to the chapter order, so let's begin with an overview of the chapters to help you decide where to start.

Chapter 1: Think

"Think" focuses on the need for critical thinking in order to navigate the multitude of health claims and contradictions we see in daily life. We look at the basic concept of healthy skepticism and the numerous errors in logic and rationality to which humans are susceptible, with the emphasis squarely on health and medical issues. By learning how to critically evaluate information, you will be better able to concentrate on behaviors that work—and not be distracted by irrelevant practices.

Chapter 2: Change

In "Change," the challenge is how to actually *do* the behaviors that have been shown to improve health. Learning ways to live better is often the easy part—the actual lifestyle modification is the true challenge. Here I review simple, tried-and-true strategies for setting goals and successfully achieving your health objectives. I also outline the psychology of change and teach you how to find your motivation, plan your strategy, and increase your chances of success.

Chapter 3: Eat

"Eat" analyzes perhaps the most complicated and confusing aspect of a healthy life: diet. We are overwhelmed with advice, suggestions, and philosophies that often contradict one another. Should we be vegetarian or go paleo? Choose a low-carb or no-carb eating plan? I present a more practical approach to eating, providing a framework that can be used in any cultural or specific diet, be it South Asian, Chinese, vegan, gluten-free, paleo, lactose-free, and so on. By focusing on the core tenets of a healthy diet, you can avoid the pitfalls and perils of the food and diet industries and simply eat well.

What about Weight Loss?

While evidence clearly shows that maintaining a healthy weight is extremely important in reducing health risks, I have not emphasized weight loss as a specific topic. You lose weight and prevent weight gain as a result of specific *actions*—primarily dietary choices and, to some extent, activity—which are discussed in detail. If weight loss is your goal, then this book will help you get there by showing you strategic and practical steps to achieve that objective. If you are significantly overweight, suffer from some of the potential medical consequences of being overweight (diabetes, cardiovascular disease, osteoarthritis, high blood pressure, back pain, or shortness of breath, for example), you may require more assistance. Consult your physician to discuss medically supervised diets, medication, or bariatric surgery. It is also worth remembering that being healthy is more than being slim—and that it is possible to improve your health dramatically without losing a pound.

Chapter 4: Move

"Move" focuses on activity and exercise. I explain the difference between the two as well as their numerous benefits. Spoiler alert: there is no one magic exercise, video, tool, or piece of equipment that will get you "ripped." I offer exercise advice and goal-setting strategies that are specific, practical, and designed to help all individuals become healthier—without, thankfully, having to develop a six-pack, do a triathlon, or bench-press your bodyweight. If you can increase your fitness level by any degree, you will improve your health significantly, so finding ways to do so is definitely worth the effort.

Chapter 5: Sleep

"Sleep" describes proper sleep hygiene along with specific behavioral strategies to help you deal with common sleep issues. Fatigue and lack of quality sleep are some of the most common reasons for visits to a physician. Sleeping pills and sleep aids are commonly prescribed and used by patients despite the lack of great evidence of their effectiveness, plus their strong side effects and risks. For many of you, sleeping better at night may be one of the most valuable ways to improve your health and your happiness. This chapter outlines concrete ways you can target this important, and often neglected, aspect of health.

Chapter 6: Enjoy

"Enjoy" focuses on mental health and how to increase the joy in your life. Happiness is not just the absence of depression; an increasing body of evidence proves that the feeling can be developed. This chapter outlines effective strategies to enjoy life and *be happier*. I discuss the concepts of purpose, gratitude, and flow, along with other practical techniques to increase your satisfaction and contentedness. Being happy is an important goal for all of us (more common than aspiring for money and fame), and it is reassuring to know that there are things you can do to improve your mental health, which in turn can pay huge dividends for your physical health.

Chapter 7: Quit

"Quit," simply put, is about quitting smoking. If you don't smoke, keep it that way. If you currently smoke, putting the effort into quitting will be the best thing you can do for your health. People often spend incredible amounts of time, effort, and money on other aspects of wellness without targeting this one issue that has the most immediate and negative impact on their health. In this chapter, I provide smokers with practical tips and motivation to help them quit and provide nonsmokers with the tools and understanding to encourage friends and loved ones to free themselves from tobacco addiction.

Chapter 8: Vaccinate

No single health intervention has been more effective from a truly preventive aspect than vaccinations (excluding handwashing and the development of a sewer system). However, we are seeing a vocal minority speak against them, which is causing a higher risk of potentially lethal illnesses making a comeback. When there is confusion and an illusion of danger, it is understandable that some parents and individuals are hesitant. Unfortunately, this feeling of uncertainty commonly leads families to not vaccinate, which should concern us all. Simply put, vaccines are safe and they work. "Vaccinate" reviews the evidence and addresses the myths and concerns that people commonly express surrounding vaccinations. Hopefully, once you understand the science, the only hurdle will be updating your immunization status.

Chapter 9: Screen

"Screen" addresses another aspect of preventive health: detecting disease when it is more treatable. While some screening programs are effective in picking up conditions early and can make a difference in outcomes, only a few diseases are truly amenable to this strategy. Unfortunately, we are just not able to effectively screen for every condition or cancer out there. Given the confusion around these limitations, I outline the criteria required to make screening a viable option and identify which programs are currently recommended. I also review the potential challenges and dangers of screening and over-testing in general.

Chapter 10: Supplement?

When people picture healthy living, they often imagine they have to supplement their life with numerous vitamins and concoctions. This final chapter, "Supplement?," questions the role of a supplement—it should be *in addition to* the strategies for health outlined earlier. If the previous nine factors are not being employed to their fullest, then the potential benefit any supplemental product or treatment provides is minimal compared to the proven benefits of the other actions. Safety, cost, and plausibility should also be factored in when considering unproven therapies. In this chapter, I teach you how to decide if taking a supplement makes sense for you.

While I strongly believe in the techniques and evidence outlined here, I must emphasize that my way is not the only way; I do not believe there is one true path to achieving health. My hope is to outline the main categories in which to focus your efforts in order to improve your chances of having a long and healthy life. While the suggestions are specific, what they will look like in real life will depend on you, the reader. *This is your life and your health* and it is up to you to find your own route to wellness.

All you can do is control what you can and give yourself the best chance to be healthy. I know people like and want guarantees, but life is full of uncertainty; we need to accept that and understand that we can only control so much. Thankfully, even though it seems like illness is commonplace, we are actually healthier than ever before. I strongly believe that reaching your eighties with minimal disability is a reasonable and attainable goal. That's my objective—but if it doesn't happen, I'll roll with it, knowing that I've done what I can and am still enjoying my life fully. After all, the aim is to live a long and *enjoyable* life, not to suffer and restrict ourselves so that life just seems long!

My hope is that after reading this book you will be motivated and energized to find areas of your life that you can improve, and you find joy and contentment in the life you are currently living.

Disclaimer

While this book does provide advice on your health, it is not meant to replace the guidance of your own physician. Hopefully this resource can augment and supplement the care you are currently receiving. At no point do I advise stopping any medications, so do not consider doing that without first talking to your doctor. If you have any health problems or symptoms that cause you concern, please contact your physician for assessment.

One final note around language—I use the term "doctor," "physician," and "primary care provider" to refer to the person responsible for the care of a patient. This is for ease of use; I certainly respect the role that other providers may play in providing this care, including nurses, nurse practitioners, and physician assistants. I respect and value all members of the health-care team in their roles to provide high-quality primary care.

1

Think

"Knowing a great deal is not the same as being smart;
intelligence is not information alone but also judgment, the
manner in which information is collected and used."
Carl Sagan

AFTER I GRADUATED from medical school, completed my residency, and began my family medicine practice, I considered myself a well-educated person who was versed in critical thinking. I had done well in school, felt I was up-to-date on health matters, and was ready to deal with the various issues that would be presented to me as a primary care practitioner.

Then I met my wife, Andrea, and we had our first child...

We began our life together just outside of Vancouver, BC, where there is a thriving and accepted culture of alternative therapies. Vancouver is kind of like California in how it has embraced "complementary" interventions. It is neither uncommon nor surprising for people to look for health-care alternatives when they are an accepted option in society. My wife was open to and interested in some of these modalities.

Her mother had recently passed away from leukemia, and we had experienced a couple of miscarriages before we had our first of two boys. Andrea then became a new mother with all the worries and anxieties that entails. She is also a healthy and active woman who desires to stay that way.

Add to these factors the honest yet really unsatisfactory answers you receive when asking many challenging health questions to medical doctors and it's easy to see why people are looking for alternative therapies.

"Why did my mother get leukemia?"
"We don't know. Bad things just happen sometimes."

"Why am I having miscarriages?"
"We don't know. Older eggs, most likely. It's common and doesn't mean you won't be successful. Keep trying."

"How can I stay healthy for the long term now that I am a parent?"
"Just keep doing what you're doing."

I had my misgivings about Andrea's interest in these therapies, but I love my wife and felt there was no harm in the occasional appointments she attended or comments she might make about diet or certain modalities, like acupuncture, Chinese medicine, or craniosacral therapy. I was even open to hearing about these options, as they were commonly brought up by my patients. After all, it is incredibly easy for alternative medicine to creep into daily life with the rise of so many pseudoscientific practices.

I thought I was a progressive physician: nonjudgmental and open to anything that could be of benefit. Then, in the course of my practice, some specific experiences really made me question this philosophy, take a hard look at my thought processes, and question how safe some of these practices were. I saw patients who:

- delayed appropriate medical care for serious illnesses while they were being treated by alternative practitioners;

- received treatment for newborns and infants for nonexistent trauma related to the natural process of childbirth;

- received poor and dangerous medical advice regarding medications, vaccinations, or specific conditions while they were being treated by alternative health practitioners for other issues;

- missed their last Christmas with their family as they were receiving ineffective alternative treatment for an unfortunately devastating and universally terminal illness; and

- suffered lifelong developmental damage due to an illness that is preventable with vaccination.

These experiences really shook me, frustrated me, and forced me to analyze my entire outlook. They also made me realize I had to do better when handling my patients' concerns about the value of various products and activities. In some ways, these discussions are about more than a specific alternative treatment modality or supplement; we are addressing and challenging someone's *worldview*. Some believe that these complementary treatments offer a valid alternative to what "Western" medicine can provide, or, perhaps understandably, look elsewhere when medicine has little to offer or appears to have failed them.

But just because science and medicine lack all the answers, it doesn't mean that alternatives are automatically valid. As the saying goes, just because airline travel isn't perfect, it doesn't mean we should start using magic carpets. The same is true for medicine. It all comes down to the old joke: *What do you call complementary or alternative medical therapies that work? Medicine.* Doctors are equal opportunity providers:

if a treatment is proven to work, we are more than happy to recommend it.

I am incredibly grateful that my wife is an open, honest, and intelligent woman who was interested in having this conversation and was willing to hear my points of view. After careful analysis and honest discussion, Andrea was able to see the rationale behind my concerns about these therapies. Without her, I likely wouldn't have been forced to analyze my own weaknesses in critical thinking. And without her, I wouldn't have so carefully researched how to be better at evaluating information and how to present that perspective to someone with a different viewpoint.

What Is Critical Thinking and Why Is It Important?

When I first started looking at the subject of critical thinking, I was amazed at how often our weaknesses in this area are routinely taken advantage of, particularly in the world of advertising. Every commercial is trying to sell you something based on some sort of association with a celebrity, a song, a joke, a model, or a movie, the logic of which quickly breaks down with basic analysis. Yet it must work, as companies continue to spend huge amounts of money on these campaigns.

Critical thinking is simply the process of analyzing a topic objectively prior to forming a judgment on that issue, opposed to simply going by your instincts or your "gut." In order to do this, you need to be aware of what may be influencing those feelings, including common *biases*—preconceived ideas that aren't based on sound reason—and *errors in logic* that all humans make when thinking about a subject. But because it takes effort, our thinking is easily manipulated by media, advertisers, and even our friends and colleagues.

Our education systems tend to inadequately prepare us to handle and evaluate the sheer onslaught of information to which we are continually exposed. We are taught facts but rarely asked to question them or their sources. Every day we are exposed to claim after claim about health. How do we know what to believe? What makes someone an "expert"? When do we believe an "expert" opinion and when do we dig deeper? How deep do we need to go? I mean, who has the time to research every paper referenced in a magazine article or question every claim made in a thirty-second commercial?

Thankfully, by being aware of the common tricks and methods used, you can ignore the irrelevant information and focus on the important stuff. That is why I believe critical thinking is the first step toward a healthy lifestyle. It allows you to concentrate your efforts on the areas that make the difference for your health and thoughtfully disregard those areas that can take you off course.

While critical thinking is a huge topic in and of itself, my goal here is simply to introduce a basic strategy so you can analyze any health claim. This chapter is not meant to tell you *what* to think but rather to outline a process for *how* to think. After that, you can make your own conclusions. Critical thinking may force you to challenge some of your deeply held beliefs, which can be uncomfortable, but the final decision is always up to you. This chapter teaches you how to be more conscious of how your mind works; be aware of the ways you can be fooled, confused, and tricked; and feel confident in assessing any health assertion—even those in this book.

So when someone tells you about the next great health product, diet, medication, or superfood, how do you determine if those claims are valid?

Step 1: Focus on the Claim Itself

When looking at any health claim, it is important to first be very clear on *what the actual claim is*. Oftentimes, there is only a vague promise of it being "good for you." It is essential that we clarify what that promise is: Will it prolong your life? Will it reduce your risk of hospitalization or serious illness? Will it make you feel better? Will you have less pain? Only when you know the specifics of the claim can you effectively evaluate it.

Once you are clear on what is specifically being offered, it is essential to keep the focus on the idea or product itself and not on the individual offering it. While controversial issues can cause an emotional response (just look at the comments section of a story on vaccines or politics), the best way to maintain civility is to emphasize the concept, which is always fair game for debate, and not the individual endorsing it.

A genius can hold an absolutely absurd position and a fool can say something profound, so using the source of a claim as a reason to believe or disbelieve something is not logically sound. For example, any advertisement featuring a well-toned celebrity is using that person's identity/appearance/fitness/movie character as a basis for recommending the product or treatment. Just because someone plays a superhero in a movie does not make their recommendation to use a product or treatment valid. And though most physicians are pretty skeptical of anything Dr. Oz recommends, that does not mean that there is nothing of value in any of the actions or products he promotes. Bottom line: the attributes of the person making the claim have nothing to do with the validity of the claim itself. There needs to be scientific basis and support for an idea, and the opinion of any individual isn't enough.

Most importantly, for the purposes of civility in discussion, it is crucial to avoid *attacking* a person making the claim rather than talking about the assertion itself. While personal attacks can feel temporarily satisfying from a sense of superiority, they are not appropriate, intellectually sound, or kind. The key is to offset our inherent tendency to concentrate on who makes a claim and instead focus on the statement itself.

Step 2: Determine the Pre-test Probability

Today, everything seems to have evidence behind it. "Studies show" different vitamins, procedures, or health devices to be effective. Before analyzing each study in detail, it is important to think about one specific aspect of the claim itself: What is the likelihood that the claim is true even before looking at the results or data? How does our knowledge of the world currently, and the existing body of science, influence the probability that this statement is true? This process of thinking can be considered as the *pre-test probability* for the intervention.

For example, one of the simpler health interventions is homeopathy. This is the belief that "like cures like"—a substance that could harm a human in normal doses can be helpful in tiny doses. In actuality, the dose is diluted to such an incredible extent that there is sometimes *literally nothing* in the homeopathic product other than water. The resulting justification is that the *water holds the memory of the substance* and thus is still effective—which makes you wonder how water-treatment plants can effectively allow us to reuse our waste water. This surprising concept is behind all those homeopathic items at the drugstore.

So in this case, the pre-test probability that a vial of plain water is able to cure or treat anything is essentially zero—given what we know about science, water, health, and how the body works. When the occasional study suggests a homeopathic item is effective, it is much more likely due to chance or error rather than the effect of the product. It would take an incredible number of high-quality studies to change the established understanding on this type of therapy.

If someone tells me I would benefit from eating more fruits and vegetables, which would seem pretty reasonable to me given what we already know about health and nutrition, I would accept that quite easily. But if they said I need to significantly increase my intake of whale fat to achieve optimal health, I would be pretty skeptical from the start. In an even simpler nonmedical example, I would easily believe someone who said they saw a squirrel in their backyard, but it would take a heck of a lot of evidence to believe them if they said they saw Bigfoot.

"Studies" are not enough anymore; they need to be high quality, reputable, repeatable, and consistent with our current body of knowledge. Science-based health advice should be our standard beyond simple "evidence." Keeping the pre-test probability in mind, especially when considering the basic building blocks of health, will allow you to discard many frivolous health claims right from the start and focus on what actually works.

Step 3: Check for Biases

As stated earlier, a cognitive bias is any idea or opinion that is preconceived or not based on sound reason. These biases can strongly influence how you see and analyze data even before you start looking at the information; by definition, you are not even aware of them. Your best defense is to bring these biases to the surface and make conscious choices to rationally evaluate them. It can be uncomfortable and unsettling, but that's a sign that you are challenging one of your built-in biases.

One of our more common tendencies is to seek out and remember things that support what we already think, while avoiding information that is contrary to what we believe. Imagine you strongly believe that vaccines are dangerous. You are presented with two articles: one by a fellow vaccine skeptic who outlines further reasons to support this viewpoint, and the other by a medical doctor who clearly states the reasons why vaccines are safe and why your viewpoint is wrong. Which article would you be more likely to read?

Repeated studies show that you would be much more likely to read the article that agrees with what you already think. We see this consistently in the way we read articles pertaining to health, the environment, and politics. This bias is exacerbated online where algorithms are used to provide you with more articles similar to the ones that you have already read, so you will be exposed to more and more support for what you already think— even if it is wrong. This happens to such an extent that two neighbors with opposing views on politics or the environment can have very little overlap in the news and articles they read.

It is therefore up to you to occasionally seek out the contrary point of view—challenging psychologically, but critical intellectually. To be clear, seeking the alternative viewpoint does not mean that you have to weigh all information equally. The opinion of an expert on immunization who has studied extensively and works exclusively in the field of vaccinations should be valued much more than the opinion of a blogger. You need to review other points of view, but you also need to be able to weigh the value of that information.

Another form of bias was uniquely demonstrated by a mathematician during World War II. Abraham Wald was a Hungarian-born Jewish statistician who fled Europe and helped the US military. When providing advice on where to best place the limited armor available on military planes to increase the chance of them surviving a battle, he looked at the locations of bullet holes on returning planes. He realized that you should actually put more armor where you see less damage, as the planes that were hit in those areas were less likely to have made it back, whereas the locations with more hits were more survivable. Clearly, you can't make your decision based on only the planes that returned—you also have to consider that ones that did not come back.

A simple health example is when people mention their friend or relative who smoked all their life and had no major health issues, using this as justification that the risk is lower than we think. Obviously, they are disregarding all the other people who smoked all their lives who developed lung problems and did not make it past seventy.

A conflict of interest—where an individual receives personal benefit or gain from promoting a particular product or viewpoint—is also important to consider when creating context for assessing any health claim. While this may not be a true cognitive bias, it is something to keep in mind when considering the point of view of someone promoting a particular idea.

I understand the skepticism people might have about me, a medical doctor writing a book and promoting a particular viewpoint on health. I also understand the concerns around the medical relationship with pharmaceutical companies and the idea that we are all "pill pushers." However, I do not get directly paid by anyone to write a prescription and in Canada the rules have thankfully changed to prevent any undue gifts given to doctors by drug companies. I don't believe they are even allowed to give out pens anymore. (I'm not sure on that, as I made the choice a number of years ago to stop seeing pharmaceutical representatives in my office.)

In contrast to the immense pushback (often rightly so) against doctors' prescribing practices, I am amazed that people are not disturbed by the direct conflict of interest seen in offices where vitamins and other health products are overtly sold. If you see a health professional who sells supplements directly to their clients as part of their business, what is the likelihood that you won't be recommended to buy something?

Being aware of potential conflicts is certainly an important aspect of assessing any health claim to provide *context*, but it should be secondary to the actual concept being considered. Just because the person selling the product believes in it does not mean that the idea is wrong—but you should be aware that the relationship can create an unconscious bias.

Above all, critical thinking needs to be objective and rational—and not personal. Think of the pre-test probability, focus on the claim, and try to bring awareness to any potential biases at play. After that, you can look at the actual foundation behind the assertion.

Step 4: Assess the Basis of the Claim

Rather than getting into the details of analyzing studies (which is impractical for most people to do), I want to instead focus on highlighting the many common—and faulty—arguments for health claims. There are weak foundations behind many of our decisions about health. By making these errors in reasoning conscious, instead of subconscious, we can realize how and when our thinking goes awry. We can then learn how to make better decisions based on objective thinking. These logical fallacies are inherent in all of us, so it is up to us to overcome them and not be fooled as easily.

Anecdotes Do Not Equal Data

One of the most common marketing techniques when it comes to medical treatments and therapies is that of the testimonial, which is just an anecdote—a specific incident or story that is used as evidence. In the sales world, an individual describes how effective the treatment was for him or her, and you are then supposed to accept that as fact and proof for the claims at hand.

Leaving aside the likelihood that many said testimonials may well be false and are used to mislead the public, even true ones should be taken with caution, if at all. Anecdotes are the worst and weakest form of evidence: there is no way to confirm them, and there are no controls in place to ensure the treatment is the actual cause for the improvement.

For example, almost all fitness-related claims are full of anecdotes and before/after pictures; however, it is never exactly clear what else the testifiers have done to achieve their results—most commonly, a highly restricted diet on top of the workout plan or device.

Even medical professionals can be easily swayed by personal stories. I recall a colleague saying that one of the worst justifications for doing anything is "In my experience..." We are understandably influenced by our experiences and so we must be extra vigilant to not be tricked by ourselves. For example, I could prescribe a drug that has a known rare side effect but also offers significant proven benefits. If my patient was unlucky enough to experience that side effect, I need to understand that the side effect will not happen to every patient, and that it is prudent to continue to prescribe that medication, for the appropriate patient with appropriate counseling, if the circumstances warrant it. I can't let my experience of witnessing the side effect make me afraid and then do the wrong thing for all future patients.

Likewise, if I have a patient who takes some supplement and swears that it helped her with her arthritis or diarrhea or whatever, I shouldn't start immediately recommending that product over traditional evidence-based treatments, without at least first reviewing the scientific evidence.

Anecdotes need not be discounted, but we must realize that they are a really weak form of evidence that, if anything, may prompt further research and study of the intervention.

One Thing Leads to Another

Another reason we often think that something we've tried is effective is because one thing happens *after* another. It does not mean that the latter was *caused* by the former.

This method of thought is the common basis for superstitions and magical thinking. For example, "My team won the baseball game when I wore this T-shirt, so I'm going to wear the same T-shirt for every game from now on (and not even wash it)!" This is an obvious case where clearly the T-shirt had nothing to do with the outcome of the game, but there are many cases where the circumstances are not as obvious.

Oftentimes, people will use multiple health interventions at the same time and assume that one in particular was the cause for improvement, despite many other potential reasons for it. For example, a person may feel the turmeric he took for the past month helped shrink his tumor but disregard the chemotherapy he received earlier, which may take some time to take effect.

There are also many conditions that improve on their own, and the intervention had nothing to do with it. In my practice as a family physician, many patients request antibiotics for viral illnesses because they are convinced that they always get better when they take an antibiotic for their bad colds. However, the natural course of a cold is to get better over time. The patient would have improved with or without the antibiotics, which kill *bacteria* but do nothing to fight viruses. One had nothing to do with the other.

Regression to the Mean

Any health condition, particularly a chronic one, tends to have a fluctuating course where there are good days and bad. For example, if you have chronic back pain, there will be days when you feel fairly good and are able to do more, and there will be days when your pain is worse and you are more limited. On which days do you think you are more likely to seek treatment? On the bad days, of course.

When a patient takes a medication on their bad days, it is hard to know if the treatment is helping or if it is the natural course of their condition with its normal pattern of ups and downs. This difference is very challenging to detect individually, which is why carefully controlled studies are required to see if medications truly work.

This phenomenon is called regression to the mean, where things will settle into their regular, or average, state over time—whether it is the level of pain a patient experiences, the percentage of free throws a basketball player makes, or the percentage of times a flipped coin turns up heads. This factor is involved in our next topic of discussion.

Placebo Effect

Any drug, supplement, or treatment has the potential to cause a placebo effect—the real decrease of symptoms of a condition or disease but one that is not due to the intervention itself. Because of the profound nature of this response, any medical trial has to account for the placebo effect to prove that the medication is truly beneficial.

With alternative medicine, the placebo effect is the main mechanism by which people feel a positive effect. By definition, if the treatment or product has been proven to work better than a placebo (a substance that is known to have no therapeutic benefit), it would no longer be called "alternative medicine," it would simply be "medicine."

Some of the manual (hands-on) therapies that have not been able to show clear benefit—despite multiple studies—can be seen as really good examples of how to optimize the placebo effect. Acupuncture therapy, for example, does not fit with what we know about how the body works but is rather based on the belief of the existence of meridians in the body and the use of needles to help increase or decrease the flow of chi (or energy) through these meridians.

Imagine you are the client who is seen by someone who you feel is a reputable practitioner, who really cares about you, and truly believes in what they're doing. This person then spends some time discussing your health and life with you (and who doesn't like thinking and talking about themselves and their priorities for a while during their hectic lives?). They then give you a clear, specific, and confident explanation for the cause of your symptoms (whether accurate or not) and explain how the treatment will address this underlying issue (again, whether accurate or not). Next, you are prepared and positioned—often in a warm room with a heating pad and soothing music. The needles are inserted, which is a physical, noticeable treatment you can clearly feel. Combine this experience with the fact that you have paid for this service and are thus motivated to have it work, and you have a terrific recipe for maximizing the placebo effect.

There are many great books on this topic and one I recommend is *Snake Oil Science* by R. Barker Bausell, which clearly outlines how the placebo effect, as well as the logical, psychological, and physiologic errors inherent in humanity, perpetuates the idea that many treatments are effective when, in reality, they are not.

The Ancient Fallacy

Another common rationale for justifying a particular treatment is that it has been around forever and was used by ancient cultures or civilizations. I'm sure you've all heard some version of the following:

"Acupuncture has been around for thousands of years, so it must be effective."

"I hear you have some kidney trouble. You should try this herbal product—it's been used in China forever."

"Ayurvedic massage has been used for millennia in India for rheumatological conditions—I'm sure it will help you too."

But I bet you haven't heard any of these:

"Are you still getting those headaches? You should see my guy—he will drill a hole in your head and take that pressure away. It was the treatment of choice for hundreds of years!"

"Clearly your infection needs to be treated by the age-old technique of bleeding. It's one of the oldest medical treatments known to man."

"One of the best ways to treat your increased family history of cancer is human sacrifice—it's been used forever!"

Clearly, I'm being over-the-top with these examples, but the fallacy is the same. Just because something is old does not mean it is good, safe, or effective. These treatments were developed and promoted in a world that predates science, cell theory, and germ theory before the concepts of bacteria, viruses, handwashing, or human anatomy were understood. The practitioners had no idea how or why a treatment would work, so they would create their own story to explain the mechanism of action.

Science can be, and has been, used to test these claims and some old herbal remedies or treatments have been found to have some mild benefit. However, just because some ancient methods have been shown to be somewhat effective and there is some explanation for effect, that does not mean that every ancient treatment is good. Those that have been shown to have merit are more a testament to the value of the scientific method than that of the ancient fallacy. So, the next time you hear someone promote a practice based on that of a wise and ancient culture, ask for their thoughts on bleeding and human sacrifice as well.

Appeal to Nature

Many people believe that simply because something is natural, it is inherently good. This argument often comes into play when discussing herbal remedies over pharmaceutical medications.

There are many herbal substances that have a physiological effect and have been used to create and develop medications (digoxin from the foxglove plant, antibiotics from molds, etc.). The idea that all things natural are safe, however, is a large leap from the idea that some substances may have benefit. Simple examples of natural things that aren't exactly safe include poison ivy, curare poison, arsenic, and poisonous mushrooms.

In considering the appeal to nature, we can acknowledge that there is value to eating whole foods and getting outside into nature, but also be aware that there is a danger in believing that if something is natural it is therefore safe and better than the alternative. In addition, as I often tell my patients, if a natural product has any *effect* at all, then it must also have the potential for *side effects* just as any drug does. The body doesn't know or care about the source of the medication.

Credibility of Studies

While I do not want to get too deep into the analysis of scientific studies, I do want to briefly comment on what to look for when you hear or read about a study. Often media and research institutes overplay the value of the results of their work in order to get attention for their work or university. Some things to watch out for include:

- *Basic science studies.* A petri dish in a laboratory is not the same thing as a human being. It is a large step from showing positive results in a basic science lab to showing similar effects in people. It is best to ignore those results and not make any health decisions based on dramatic headlines stemming from this type of study.

- *Animal studies.* Mice are not human beings, and very few studies on animals end up showing similar results in people or even get to the point of being studied in humans. Ignore any exciting headlines regarding cures for cancer if the study population was a group of rats or some other non-human animal.

- *The quality of studies.* Look for high-quality studies that have been randomized, have control groups to account for the placebo effect, are double-blind (participants and investigators don't know who is receiving the study drug/intervention), have lots of study subjects, and are published in high-quality journals. As stated previously, all manner of health interventions appear to have some sort of evidence behind them, so it is worth considering the quality of the human studies.

While that is probably more information than you need when considering evidence presented in the media, it is worthwhile to keep these factors in mind when thinking about all the health claims you are exposed to. The bottom line is that if any dramatic discovery is clearly proven to markedly improve health, it will have to have gone through a significant process to get there—and you will be unlikely to miss it. Until then, you should be skeptical of the claims you hear, particularly in regards to the fundamental factors of a healthy life that are unlikely to change significantly.

Heuristics: What Prevents Us from Thinking Critically?

As demonstrated, we humans regularly make errors, have biases, and jump to conclusions, naturally leading to the question, "Why are we so bad at analyzing information?" The answer is that we actually aren't; we are very good at making quick decisions on straightforward matters. The issues arise when we look at more complex ones.

A significant problem is that the logical fallacies mentioned above are actually effective in many situations—that is why they developed and persist. They are based on heuristics, which are any techniques, processes, or methods that are used to find solutions to problems. Some typical types of heuristics are trial and error, educated guesses, and rules of thumb. These are obviously better than the alternative of brute force, where one considers every potential solution equally, and random guesses, but they do not ensure the discovery of the right answer.

In many circumstances, however, those errors in logic actually serve a purpose. As a parent, I like to use my role as their father to convince my children ("Don't argue with me! Just do what I say... I'm your father!"). As our children have started to understand and learn the importance of being able to defend and support any claims they make, this argument unfortunately no longer works—I only have myself to blame. However, in some situations, such as where safety is involved (yelling "Stop!" when walking near traffic, for example), it may be best for our children to just trust their loving parents and do what we say.

Now that we aren't helpless children, why do we continue to use these heuristics and not think for ourselves? Simply put: they are much quicker and easier than the alternative. In terms of health information, it would be exhausting to fully analyze every claim we hear—it is easier to use our tried-and-true heuristics and just trust them. So, often we pick an outlook that is supported by our experience or shared by someone we trust ("natural is better" or "Big Pharma can't be trusted") and rely on it in our decision-making. Again, perfectly understandable, but it does not result in us making reliably good assessments.

What heuristics do, however, is provide us with a framework to have some certainty in how we see the world. They give us security and comfort. Unfortunately, many of the issues we deal with (science, health, politics, and the environment) are complicated, and simply wishing something to be black or white does not make it so.

One heuristic or mental shortcut that I believe could be useful in regards to general health is to focus on the ten basic components of healthy living outlined in this book and downplay the rest until or unless there is a clear reason to do so. Given what we know about how the human body works, and the huge body of scientific research we have in these areas, any benefit claimed from a superfood or a terrific medication will likely be small compared to the huge value in focusing on an overall healthy diet, increasing physical activity, or sleeping better. But I hope you come to believe this not because I said so as a medical doctor, but because the suggestions make sense in their own right and resonate with you.

Science and medicine, in particular, do not tend to be intuitive. We can be easily fooled, with all of those simple heuristics, or educated guesses, quickly leading to wrong conclusions. That is why science and critical thinking are such powerful tools, as systems to minimize bias, test ideas, and get results that either support or oppose them. Science actively works to expose errors in our heuristics and creates theories that can be fine-tuned and truly relied upon.

I love how Carl Sagan describes science in the subtitle of his great book *The Demon-Haunted World*: "Science as a Candle in the Dark" which is a wonderful tribute to reason and a warning of what can happen if we allow ourselves to stop thinking critically—a return to darkness. We may have had an excuse in the prescientific world, but in the twenty-first century that excuse is no longer valid. We need to continue to move toward further understanding of our amazing universe and continue to illuminate our world.

Summary

Using your rational thoughts to evaluate and consider your many choices around wellness is an essential component to leading a healthy life. We humans are easily fooled—particularly when it comes to health. Understand how and why you tend to think the way you do and learn ways to combat your own errors in reasoning through critical thinking.

You can feel confident that you are doing this, and being rational in evaluating health claims, by using a consistent process:

1. Focus on the claim itself.
2. Determine the pre-test probability.

3. Check for biases.
4. Assess the basis of the claim.

Knowledge is power; by understanding these basic steps to analyze information and identify common errors in critical thinking, it may be hard to blindly accept advice again—and that's a good thing. Build your skills in critical thinking so that when you hear a health claim that you want to consider—including those in this book—you can use reason to assess it.

2

Change

"Only I can change my life. No one can do it for me."
Carol Burnett

IN MY MEDICAL practice, I see patients every day who are struggling with their health and clearly want to make some changes to improve their lives. Often it is very easy to find areas to improve—eating better, exercising more, sleeping more, watching less television, drinking less alcohol, quitting smoking, drinking less soda, and so on...

Despite these many options, often no changes have been made by the time I see them again. The desire to make change is there, the knowledge of what to change is there, yet the *ability* to change seems to be lacking. Patients want to be healthier and know lots of techniques to help them achieve that goal, so *why don't they do them?*

The simple reality is that change is hard—especially when talking about the daily habits that influence our health. These typically aren't one-time fixes, like choosing to use skim milk instead of whole milk (although that can be important too), but rather pervasive habits that have been ingrained in us.

They require not just simple change but a dramatic lifestyle modification.

In most cases, this change doesn't seem to happen until the patient finds their inner motivation (a personal health scare, a family health issue, a new baby) and then truly feels the need to transform. There are lots of other reasons we struggle with change as well.

- We don't really want to stop the things that are bad for us: *"I know I should quit smoking but I just like it too much!"*

- We aren't specific enough with our goals: *"I'm going to start eating better."* Whatever that means...

- We are spoiled for choice and can't decide what to focus on, so we don't do anything: *"My doctor says I need to start walking, quit smoking, lose fifty pounds, stop drinking soda, drink less alcohol, and go to bed earlier... Ah, forget it!"*

- We set our sights too high, become dejected, and give up: *"I haven't done any exercise for years so I signed up to run a half-marathon next month."*

- We don't really believe in, care about, or even have a true reason to change: *"My doctor says I need to change my lifestyle so I don't have a heart attack, but my parents were way worse than me and they lived well into their eighties..."*

Given such issues, it is absolutely understandable that lifestyle change as a means of improving health is hard. I bet you're a bit like me in that you have great intentions and desires to make more positive changes, but the reality of making them happen is a challenge. In addition to personally wanting to continually improve my own health, I am also involved with the day-to-day work of motivating patients in theirs, as well as motivating physicians to improve their practices. As a result, I understand how difficult it is to find motivation to make alterations in how we live and work. Thankfully, there has been lots of research regarding change management and how to best handle the challenges involved.

Numerous factors are involved in any lifestyle modification strategy, and although it is hard to change fundamental behaviors, it is certainly doable. In this chapter, we review several practical concepts to create a specific change strategy that is useful, pertinent, and realistic. This individualized approach can then be used to help achieve whichever health goal you are willing to work toward—possibly one addressed in a subsequent chapter.

Be the Dictator of Your Health

When it comes to your personal health, you are the only one who can determine the best reasons for making changes, which specific area(s) in your life you want to address, and what specific types of modifications you are willing and able to make. Your healthcare provider or friend or fitness consultant can give you some ideas, but it is up to you to make the final decisions and take action. No one else can do this work for you.

Making this decision may seem daunting at first, but it is also freeing and simple. When you know it is up to you, there are no excuses or finger-pointing to hold you back. An interesting story to exemplify this resolve involves the zoologist Alan Rabinowitz, founder of Panthera, a nonprofit organization dedicated to protecting the world's forty wild cat species.

Rabinowitz grew up with a severe stutter and struggled mightily to communicate. As a child, he avoided speaking in public even to the point that he stabbed his hand with a pencil in order to avoid having to answer a question in class. Eventually he found some solace in talking to his pets; he was able to speak full sentences to them and appreciated their lack of judgment. Rabinowitz realized that they were like him in that they didn't have a voice, so he promised that he would act as the voice for animals: this became his motivation and his passion.

Rabinowitz's story is fascinating and inspiring on many levels, but what I feel relates to this section most is his take on the challenge of working with dictators and other leaders of countries where big cats are most at risk. He said that in many ways it was easier dealing with a dictator than with a democratic government since he only had to convince one person and there was much less bureaucracy.

I'm not advocating for dictatorships, but the parallel in wellness is that *only you* have to make the decision to change; there are no meetings to arrange, committees to convene, or votes to lobby for. The power and ability to improve your own health rests with you and you alone. That makes it simple, straightforward, and achievable... doesn't it? Certainly, making a change is a great power, a great responsibility, and a great challenge—but who else would you want to have control over your health?

Model for Change

After reading numerous books about change, attending conferences on the challenges of transforming medical habits, and working with physicians dealing with change in their practices (when transitioning to electronic medical records or a new scheduling system), I have found one model that best demonstrates the aspects of change that need to be navigated. It is that of a rider on an elephant going down a path, which was described by University of Virginia psychologist Jonathan Haidt in his book *The Happiness Hypothesis*. Chip Heath and

Dan Heath then borrowed that analogy in their great book *Switch*—which is the one book focused on change that I most recommend—to describe in detail the three elements we have to motivate and control in our quest for change.

This analogy encompasses the major components that need to be addressed if you are to be successful in making significant change. The rider is your brain—able to understand intellectually what you need to do to improve your health and what steps to take in order to get there. The elephant represents your heart, or your deep inner motivation for becoming healthier. While the rider can decide on the direction to go, the much more powerful elephant needs to be on board with the plan or else you will have very little chance of reaching your destination.

The final element is the path that reminds you to make adjustments in your environment to make the journey easier. There are numerous challenges on your route—the ease of access to high-calorie foods, the limited time available to exercise, the pervasiveness of sitting in your job, and the constant access to technology which can affect your ability to sleep, for example. You need to clear and modify the path in order to achieve your goals.

All three of these elements need to be considered to create meaningful change, particularly in regards to healthy behaviors. By understanding them, you can focus on solutions to optimize each aspect and make your goal of improving your health more attainable. In my mind, the most important and challenging issue in regards to your well-being is finding the deep motivation for that elephant. While we often already know in general *what* we should do to be healthier (the rider), we are not clear on the *why* (the elephant). We all intellectually know many ways we could be living more healthfully, but we have to first succeed in reining in the beast by outlining the clear reasons behind wanting change.

Motivate the Elephant

When it comes to changing your health-related behaviors, you need to find the personal motivation to carry you through the many challenges along the way. That motivation should be obvious, as everyone has reasons to try to be healthy and live longer:

I want to live independently as long as I can.
I don't want to be a burden on my family.
I want to see my grandchildren grow up.
I want to have less pain.
I want to have more energy.
I want to lose weight and feel more attractive for my partner.

Unfortunately, on their own, these ideas are usually not strong enough to push us toward action.

In *The Heart of Change*, John Kotter and Dan Cohen discuss their findings from a study they conducted to try to understand how and why change happens within large organizations, which can be extrapolated to individuals. One of their conclusions was that most people believe that we are convinced to change in the following order: Analyze-Think-Change. We are presented with data regarding the proposed change; we then process the information and hopefully understand the reason to change; and then we just do it. This process may work for smaller transformations where analysis can push us in one direction or the other, and where we can be purely objective (picking the right yogurt to buy or selecting the best route to work), but it typically doesn't apply to health matters.

In regards to our health, we are talking about changing behaviors we have been doing for years and for deep-seated reasons. These are not easily changed by simple thought and analysis. Kotter and Cohen emphasize the need to *speak to the heart*—to use an emotional push toward change. The heart is the same as the elephant in the Heaths' analogy.

Instead of Analyze-Think-Change, people are motivated to make meaningful efforts by See-Feel-Change. In this scenario, you are presented with information that hits you on a personal level and that emotional impulse drives you to change. But there is nothing much more personal than one's own health, so why is it so hard to feel motivated to do the healthy behaviors?

Change certainly does occur when the right drivers are found. Oftentimes, that reason is based on fear after a significant health scare. After experiencing a heart attack, for example, people are commonly able to make profound health changes in their diet, exercise levels, and smoking patterns. Anger can also motivate people, such as those who work hard to get fit as a means of getting back at an ex-spouse. The birth of a child or grandchild and the joy that brings can induce significant positive change. Or perhaps seeing someone you know experiencing the benefits of weight loss serves as your motivation—you feel hope.

While fear is often used by the medical community as means of motivation—consider those terrible pictures on cigarette packets—it may not be the best emotion to target. Research suggests that fear and anger can motivate people but often just temporarily. I certainly see patients who are keen on going vegan after their heart attack but are usually back eating bacon a few months later (not that there is anything wrong with bacon . . . in moderation).

So how do you target those positive feelings that will motivate your elephant? Here are some suggestions on where to start.

Ignition Statement

"The most powerful weapon on Earth is the human soul on fire."
JOHN O'LEARY, author

If you want to read a book that will inspire you to find your purpose and live your best life, consider *On Fire* by John O'Leary. It's a gut-wrenching account of how the author found a way to thrive after experiencing third-degree burns over almost his entire body. At the age of nine, O'Leary accidentally blew up his family's garage and set himself on fire. All of him—on fire. His older brother put out the fire by beating him repeatedly with a rug and rolling him around on the snowy ground, despite the intense heat and the resulting burns on his own hands and arms. His eleven-year-old sister held him and told him it would be okay despite his appearance and how hot it was to even hug him. His eight-year-old sister went back into the burning building *three times* to get water to splash onto John's face, saving his face and leaving a portion of his scalp available for future skin grafts. All of these actions—of his family members, his community, and O'Leary himself—which led to him surviving and eventually finding his way in life are truly touching and motivating. He managed to find purpose and rise above immense challenges far beyond what most of us have had to overcome.

O'Leary describes something that helped and continues to help him find his way: an ignition statement. You can always go to this one statement in order to remind yourself *why* you are doing what you are doing, why you should persevere and keep giving your all on good days and bad. I have personally found it to be an excellent tool to keep me focused when things get hard. Why do you keep doing your best? How do you keep going? What is your purpose in life? Why does your work matter? Why do you matter? Why do you want to be your best and thrive? *Because...*

Because my kids look up to me.
Because my customers depend on me.
Because God loves me.
Because I am loved, I love my family, and I have something to offer to the world.
Because I matter and what I do matters to me and my loved ones.
Because life is a gift.
Because the universe is miraculous.

Your personal ignition statement is not simple to develop. It may take some time to fine-tune your own, but once you have it down, you should be able to recite it at will and regularly to keep your elephant motivated.

Thankfully, you don't need to experience an incredible challenge like enduring terrible burns to determine your own motivation for living your healthiest life. We all deserve to have our best lives; we are all worth it.

In regards to your health, if you don't have a purpose that you already feel deep inside, then you can do a simple exercise to help find it. Take out a piece of paper and write out at least ten reasons for living a long and healthy life. Don't overthink it—just write whatever comes to mind no matter how small or trivial. Now look at that list and see what truly resonates with you and if you can create a group of your most important reasons.

Here are some examples of reasons to spark your thoughts and develop a more personal list:

To feel young and have more energy.
To have less pain.
To be able to continue traveling.
To spend more time with my children and grandchildren.
To feel better about myself.

To save money on medical expenses.
To reduce risk of illness and disease.
To reduce risk of injury.
To keep doing what I love to do.

Next, take it a step further and use that list to help create your own ignition statement—that one phrase that will help you stay motivated when the going gets tough and remind you of all those specific reasons you listed to be healthy. It's the answer to those questions when you feel challenged: Why should I go exercise today? Why shouldn't I have that chocolate bar? Why don't I just stay up and watch two more episodes?

John O'Leary's statement for getting up every day—giving his absolute best to thrive in his life, despite having days of terrible pain and fatigue—is as follows: *Because God demands it, my family deserves it, and the world is starved for it.*

My goal is to keep finding time to exercise; to make healthier food choices when I'm challenged to do so; to choose to make sleep more of a priority; and to do my best every day to be a better husband, father, doctor, and person. For my ignition statement to capture this multifaceted goal, I borrowed from O'Leary's statement and tweaked it to target my personal insecurities: *Because this gift of life demands it, my family deserves it, and because I am worth it.*

Your ignition statement should speak directly to your elephant and keep you motivated through the tough times. Take some time to create your own ignition statement to clarify your personal inspiration to live a healthy life. *Why do you want to give your best each and every day? Because...*

Becoming

When I was in my twenties, I was asked one of those personality assessment questions: "What one word would you use to describe yourself?" In a brief moment of wisdom, I said, "Becoming." I would love to say this was some well-thought-out answer based on detailed self-analysis and research, but actually it came from the 1981 crime novel by Thomas Harris, *Red Dragon*, which predated his 1988 bestseller, *The Silence of the Lambs*. The main villain had the unfortunate delusion that he was Becoming (it was capitalized in the book) this evil creature, the Red Dragon. He kept using that term, and while I thought it a bit morbid in the book, I felt it was interesting as a way of describing that feeling that I was not (and still am not) finished becoming who I will be.

It turns out this idea of becoming offers a helpful outlook on health and on your life in general. Carol Dweck, a professor of psychology at Stanford University, has studied and written extensively on the concept of fixed versus growth mindsets. She discusses these thoroughly in her great book *Mindset: The New Psychology of Success*. In a fixed mindset, you feel that your traits are specific and don't change; people are either naturally good at something or they are not. Sure, you can get better and learn skills, but in this view your ultimate talent level or ability is fixed no matter how much you work at it. In a growth mindset, you feel that anyone can truly change and any ability can be improved—if given the resources, opportunities, support, and if you work hard to achieve it.

This concept is crucial when making significant lifestyle modifications for health improvement. A growth mindset helps decrease the level of intimidation around any change by helping you to expect temporary failures and setbacks: they are just a part of the process of change and improvement. Alternatively, with a fixed mindset, those same setbacks are confirmation of your predetermined traits and proof that you couldn't do it anyway. With that kind of outlook, a setback can quickly lead to giving up.

So how do you use this concept to your advantage? First, you need to be aware of the language you use when describing yourself or others. The fixed-mindset vocabulary is everywhere and it takes effort to use words to promote growth. Compare the following statements that I hear often in my clinic and that I'm sure you have all heard or used before.

Fixed Mindset	Growth Mindset
I'm a smoker.	Right now, I smoke a half-pack a day.
I'm a terrible sleeper.	I have a hard time falling asleep some nights.
I'm a sugar addict. I can't stop eating candy.	I find it hard to resist candy at times.
I don't like to exercise.	I haven't found the right exercise for me yet.

In a growth mindset, setbacks and failures are expected to occur and are part of the process of self-improvement. If you keep that outlook in mind, you can keep doing the work needed to achieve your health goals. Failure is likely on the road to success, so don't be surprised when it happens; instead plan for it, learn from it, and move on.

Direct the Rider

Now that you have a clear motivation for achieving a healthier life, you need to provide the rider some directions on how to get there. This is the rational component of our analogy that has to be given clear instructions and a destination to get you where you want to go. The strengths of the rider lie in their ability to plan, think long-term, and decide how to channel the energy of the elephant. Proper goal setting is the key here.

SMART Goals

If you have bought or been given this book, presumably one of your goals is to *be healthier*. That's great, but it doesn't give the rider well-defined instructions. In order to increase your chance of success in anything, the acronym SMART can help you create useful objectives on your way to achieving your ultimate aim. Each letter stands for a feature of a successful goal:

Specific—well-defined and clear-cut

Measurable—can easily know if the goal was done or not

Attainable—is doable; not overstretching

Relevant—related to your ultimate goal

Time-Sensitive—for a specific period of time so you can build on your success

The first feature to discuss is *specificity*. The goal has to be clear; the rider does not like ambiguity or uncertainty. Wanting to "eat better" and "exercise more" is not good enough and is not very helpful guidance. You need a detailed action that you can prepare to do. For example, you could plan on walking three times a week; better yet, you could plan on walking for fifteen minutes, three times a week. The more specific the instruction, the easier it is for the rider to follow.

Next, the goal needs to be *measurable*. This does not mean you need to use elaborate tools, a Fitbit, or a calculator; it means that you can be held accountable in terms of whether you have achieved your goal or not. Did you achieve your target of walking three times a week? Yes or no.

One of the most important features of a good objective is

that it has to be *attainable*. We often see people make bold and extravagant New Year's resolutions to run a marathon, overhaul their diet, or stop watching television—only to give up a few days later. You want to have a goal that you can realistically achieve—you should be at least 80 percent sure that you can meet your target. In fact, it is better for the goal to be too easy rather than too hard. *It is always better to build on success than plan for failure.* So, in our example, a goal to walk for even five minutes three times a week would be a perfectly valid place to start if you have been struggling to do anything at all for years. The physical activity guideline of thirty minutes of moderate intensity activity five times a week may be a good long-term goal, but it may not be SMART.

How *relevant* the goal is to your ultimate objective is the fourth feature of a SMART goal. The behavior needs to move you toward your destination. If your goals are to be healthier, feel better, improve your energy, and maybe sleep better, then increasing your physical activity level with regular walking makes perfect sense. Taking an additional multivitamin as your sole means of healthy living, unfortunately, won't get you closer to your goal. Alternatively, if you expect that only increasing your walking will lead to significant weight loss, increased musculature, and wealth, then you will also be disappointed. The behavioral change needs to be relevant and related to the desired goal.

Finally, there should be an element of *time* associated with the goal. Giving yourself a period of time to try the behavior and track your progress allows you to modify the goal, and either advance or adjust it as necessary. After four weeks, if you were able to easily meet your walking goal, you should increase the number of times per week or the length of the session for the next four weeks. Or if you found it was too difficult, then maybe reduce the frequency to twice a week or aim for a shorter duration to make it more achievable. The goal again is to build on success and create continuous cycles of improvement leading to your eventual objective.

Remember: any SMART goal should be focused on a behavior or an action. Your ultimate objective may be to lose ten pounds, but that is not a controllable action for which you can set a successful SMART goal. Weight loss can occur as a result of numerous potential behaviors, so you need to set a specific goal for the *action* that will then *lead* to your desired outcome of losing weight. Some examples include eliminating soda from your diet, having dessert only once a week, and keeping track of calories. I will provide more information on weight-loss techniques in the next chapter, "Eat."

Prepare the Initial Steps

"The journey of a thousand miles begins with one step."
LAO-TZU, philosopher

It can be daunting to decide how to begin when trying to achieve something large like losing weight, increasing your physical activity, or improving your health in general. It must be emphasized that while there is no one way to do anything, there is one way to be sure that nothing changes: *do nothing.* Maintaining the status quo will assuredly continue your health trajectory. The first step is deciding to make a change—any change.

When you decide what specific SMART goal you will be working toward, be sure to do whatever you can to *make the first literal steps as easy as possible.* If you decide to go to the gym or do yoga first thing in the morning, setting out your workout clothes the night before may be the nudge you need to get you out of bed and get started. Those first few steps are always the hardest, so scripting them clearly can give you the energy you need to keep going.

Shape the Path

Even when we have the best intentions and the best laid plans to make positive changes, it can feel like the world is conspiring against us. Why does chocolate have to be so tasty? Why are there so many great shows to watch on Netflix? Why does the sofa have to be so comfortable? Your environment can make your desired goals that much harder to achieve, and it is the focus of the final component of our analogy—the path. Are there ways you can shape your surroundings to make the path easier for the rider and the elephant to negotiate?

Willpower and Decision Fatigue

In *Willpower*, Roy F. Baumeister and John Tierney outline the evidence that willpower is like a muscle in that it can become fatigued but it can also be strengthened. In 1996, Baumeister put some college students through a somewhat cruel process that demonstrated this effect; it's often called the radish experiment.

A group of students were asked to fast before arriving for the experiment. They were then placed in a room to wait for a set period of time. This room was filled with the smell of freshly baked chocolate chip cookies and, at their tables, were bowls with pieces of chocolate, those fresh cookies, and . . . radishes.

Half of the participants were allowed to snack as they wished and did so. The other half were allowed to eat only the radishes. They were watched and many clearly struggled with the willpower to follow through on these instructions, but no one in the radish group succumbed to eating the treats.

The next stage of the experiment involved both groups moving to another room to work on geometric puzzles. They were told they were testing how clever they were but, in reality, the puzzles were not solvable. This technique is apparently a standard way to test for perseverance in the social-science world. The results were striking—those students who were able to eat as they pleased worked on the puzzles for an average of twenty minutes. (This was also the limit for a control group that fasted but were not offered any food, in case you wondered if hunger could be the cause of any difference.) In the radish group, the students gave up after only eight minutes, suggesting that their willpower was fatigued after use.

While there has been some question regarding the size of this effect, and the consistent reproducibility of it, this result does seem to make intuitive sense. In the fall, when children return to school, parents often see an increase in difficult behaviors at the end of the day—more outbursts, more tears, and more demands. In the willpower model, it makes sense as the children have had to spend the whole day controlling themselves in order to survive the classroom environment and the behavioral limits on them. When they return home, their willpower has been depleted and their lucky parents get the pleasure of handling them in this state.

Similarly, we adults can also become fatigued by making a lot of decisions each day. I'm sure you've all been in situations where, after being forced to make lots of repetitive choices (in picking items for a wedding or choosing features when doing a renovation), you get depleted toward the end and just pick the default option or "whatever." This feeling has actually been the impetus behind researchers looking into the concept of decision fatigue, and the results confirmed their intuition. In one study, car buyers were noted to choose the default option more often as they got to the end of a long list of options. Numerous successful individuals have also realized that decision-making requires energy and they want to reserve theirs for the most important decisions; Barack Obama, Steve Jobs, and Mark Zuckerberg all elected to essentially wear the same clothes daily to eliminate "what to wear to work" from their list of decisions.

My takeaway from these areas of study is that by reducing the number of times you have to use your willpower and the number of decisions you have to make, you will improve your chances of achieving your desired goals. Beyond wearing the same uniform every day, you can make other small adjustments in your environment to allow you to have fewer choices and tax your willpower less.

Further specific examples are provided in upcoming chapters, but here are some ideas to get you started. In terms of exercise, even if you get yourself to the gym, you can be exhausted and intimidated by the immense choice of workouts, machines, and stations to use. Having a specific workout clearly in mind or a trainer to guide you will improve your success rate and allow you to spend your energy on the exercise itself rather than on deciding what exercise to do. Similarly, by not purchasing soda for the house, you can eliminate the willpower needed to choose water over that sugary treat. The science behind our psychology can be used to our advantage.

Use the Power of the Pack

Another way to help shape the path is to use the strength of the herd to keep you on track. Telling someone your goals and plans may be all you need to feel accountable and keep on trying. Or maybe having a partner to do the proposed change with (quit smoking, start walking) may be a successful choice. Or perhaps joining a workout class or group and becoming part of a community involved in the healthy behavior will ensure your continued effort. Using the strength in numbers can be an extremely effective way of keeping your elephant on path and holding your rider accountable.

Develop Habits

A habit is a behavior that we do without thinking. It essentially eliminates the use of willpower or decision-making, as the brain moves on autopilot. Obviously, there are lots of examples where this can be detrimental to your health (smoking, mindlessly eating while watching television), but is it possible to use it in a positive way?

The key to any habit is the cycle where a specific cue leads to a behavior or routine that then leads to a reward. In its simplest form, you can think of various animal experiments where a certain trigger, like a bell (*the cue*), is used to prompt a mouse to press a lever (*the routine*) to then get some food (*the reward*). Our health behaviors are more complex than that, but the principles still apply.

What has been shown to be useful, particularly in helping us do things that we know are good for us, is to simply create an *action trigger* to help develop the habit. An action trigger is a conscious situational trigger that is paired with a desired action. This action trigger helps to eliminate the need to think about when to do the action, and the specificity reduces the decision-making effort and the willpower required.

In trying to create your own positive healthy behaviors, establishing your specific action triggers can greatly improve your chance of success. Here are some more examples to start the thought process around how these can be used.

While my son is at practice, I will go for a walk.
Whenever I'm on the phone at work, I will stand up and walk around.
After I drop the kids off at school, I will go to the gym.
When I wake up, I will make a protein shake for breakfast.
After I brush my teeth, I will take my medication.

Action triggers can be used to help find time to exercise, to make better choices regarding diet, and to do any behavior by pairing it with something specific. This is another example where research into human behavior can be fairly easily incorporated into our daily lives. By focusing on what has been shown to be effective, it is possible to shape your path toward better health, providing your rider and elephant a smoother journey.

Summary

We have looked at the abundant research behind managing change and how it can be used to create a plan for improving health. Altering the many behaviors that are involved in a healthy lifestyle takes work, but it is reassuring that science has given us practical tips on how to be successful.

First, you need to *motivate your elephant* and find your personal reason for improving your health. You need to see and feel the need to make these changes in your life. What is your ignition statement to inspire that elephant? You can also decrease the level of intimidation around the change by having a growth mindset, where setbacks are an expected part of the process.

Second, you need to *direct your rider* with straight-forward instructions and a clear destination. Use concrete SMART goals and small achievable behaviors that help you build on success. Script out the first few steps of those actions to make it as easy as possible to overcome the initial inertia involved in making change.

Finally, you need to do whatever you can to *shape the path* to make it more manageable: shape the environment to reduce the need for willpower and the number of decisions; use the power of the pack to keep your motivation high; and develop action triggers and habits to make the actions more routine and easier to remember.

Change can be hard—but your health is one thing that is certainly worth the effort.

3

Eat

"A diet is the smallest number of calories and the greatest amount of exercise that a patient can tolerate. A healthy lifestyle is the smallest number of calories and the greatest amount of exercise that a patient can enjoy."
from *Best Weight* by Dr. Yoni Freedhoff and Dr. Arya Sharma

"DIET" IS A loaded term that has only become more complicated over the years. We have moved from periods where humanity struggled to have enough food, to creating diets that were consistent with local and cultural environments, to the point where high caloric foods are available for purchase at any place and time. Choosing what food and how much of it to put into our bodies in order to be healthy has become an incredible challenge.

Every day in my clinic I see people who are trying to be healthy with any number of diet systems—Weight Watchers, paleo, low fat, low carb, and vegan, for example. I also see patients struggling with the consequences of obesity—osteoarthritis, diabetes, heart disease, and liver disease, to name a few. What we eat is incredibly important to our health, yet the confusion surrounding this topic is unbelievable. Is one diet the healthiest? Is one food the source of all our health woes? I don't believe so.

My intention in this chapter is to provide you with some background regarding the challenges we have with our food choices and then some general principles to consider no matter which diet you choose to follow. These tenets provide a framework and path to help navigate the complicated food world we live in.

Any talk of diet and eating has body weight as an underlying issue or concern. Your weight and waist circumference certainly are risk factors for your health overall. However, you can't simply try to lose weight; you have to focus on the specific behaviors and actions which—on the background of your genetic and social environment—determine your weight. By keeping the general framework for healthy eating in mind, you can then look at a number of specific choices that you can make, set goals for, and achieve on your path to healthy eating, healthy living, and weight loss. Any pounds that are lost will be a result of those specific actions and the amount you lose will depend on your level of change.

But should weight loss be the ultimate goal? Perhaps not. Healthy eating is but one component of a cascade of behaviors that lead to healthy living, decreased burden of disease, and increased quality of life. It is certainly possible to feel well, improve our diet, and become healthier yet still be overweight. The true goal is to eat better and aim for the healthiest weight *for you*—not to achieve any specific weight, size, or shape. Overall, I want you to be more aware of your dietary selections so that they support your well-being rather than detract from it.

Before we go any further, I have to thank Dr. Yoni Freedhoff (weight management expert, author of *The Diet Fix*, and writer of the blog *Weighty Matters*) and Dr. Arya Sharma (obesity expert, founder of the Canadian Obesity Network) for promoting and advocating for the medical profession to do a better job in dealing with weight-management issues. I also have to credit James Fell (syndicated columnist, author of *Lose It Right*, and host of the blog *Body for Wife*) for his no-nonsense, no-holds-barred attitude to lifestyle modification. Their articles, books, and posts have greatly influenced my approach to diet and weight management and, without question, have made me a better physician.

The Challenge

Obesity rates in North America and around the world are rising dramatically. In one study, the statistics showed that the number of people considered obese in the United States more than doubled from 15 percent in 1976 to 34.9 percent in 2012. This rate of obesity has immense effects on the health of our population as a whole and thus becomes a public-health issue.

There are a multitude of reasons why this is happening, and it's worth being aware of them in order to minimize their effects on us and make plans to overcome them. While we could hope that the "system" will work to change some of these factors so it's easier for us to make healthy choices, it likely won't happen soon enough to warrant waiting. In the meantime, let's look at the issues we are up against and find ways to offset them.

Increased Access to Food

Food and beverages are around us all the time. We are inundated with advertisements encouraging us to eat and consume all day long. High-calorie foods are packaged to be eaten on the go; we can consume hundreds of extra calories and hardly be aware of it. High-calorie beverages are also a constant feature of the landscape. All of these extra calories, if not burned off, will be stored in the body and lead to weight gain.

Food is also ever present in our work and play environments. Offices regularly have snacks and treats at the ready in the breakroom (and it's always somebody's birthday). Even our children are expected to have an often-sugary snack after the briefest activity. Any sporting practice or game for young children seems to involve the offering of juice boxes, popsicles, and cookies—even if they just had breakfast.

Increased Amount of Food

Portion sizes continue to grow in our culture as well. We love a bargain, and if we're getting significantly more food for a minimal cost increase, we can't seem to pass it up—even if we don't want or need that extra food. The driving force on the part of the restaurants and businesses is likely profit; the cost of the additional portion size is minimal compared to the additional cost they can charge, even with the perceived "deal" for the consumer.

These large portions also influence our portions when cooking at home. In our house, on special occasions, my wife pulls out her grandmother's old china plates to serve dinner on. It is shocking how small the plates are compared to what we're accustomed. My normal dinner plate is more in keeping with the serving platters of old. We have all gotten used to larger portions and bigger serving sizes.

So how much have our portions increased? The Centers for Disease Control and Prevention states that restaurant portion sizes are an incredible four times larger than they were in 1950. That's a huge difference and a challenge to overcome in making healthy choices.

Increased Takeout, Eating Out, and Processed Food

Due to our hectic lives, most of us are taking less time to think about and prepare food; instead, we resort to takeout, eating out, or eating processed foods at home. These foods are designed to *sell* and thus are much higher in salt, sugar, and fat—which make us want to eat more of them and more frequently.

By eating more of these kinds of foods, you give the control of portion sizes, ingredients, and caloric density to the corporations that make the food and take it away from yourself. You are abdicating your most basic health choice and giving it to those who have very little interest in what's best for your body. These companies and products are not bad or evil, but you need to be aware of the reality that their driving force is profit, not the health of the population.

While life can be busy, it is still your responsibility to make the best decisions regarding the fuel you provide your body. Unfortunately eating out regularly is not one of them. If you can minimize how frequently you eat takeout and outside the home, you remove yourself from the challenge of eating healthfully within the corporate food environment. You also gain the incredible social benefits of cooking and eating together with family and friends. This doesn't mean you can never eat out again or that cooking at home needs to be complicated, but you need to be aware that cooking at home with simple and basic ingredients will always be a better choice than eating out.

Decreased Physical Activity?

In the digital age, more of us are spending more time sitting and less time moving. Some studies have suggested that over the past fifty years, our daily energy expenditure has decreased by only 100 calories per day, while our caloric intake has gone up five times. Another study showed that, since 1980, our overall calories burned has not changed at all despite our obesity rate doubling in that same period. So, while decreased activity is an issue, it seems that the amount we eat is the larger factor and should be the main focus if weight loss is your goal.

Certainly, I do not mean to diminish the role of exercise and activity in living a healthy lifestyle and in helping to maintain a healthy weight. In fact, some studies suggest that low cardiovascular fitness may actually be a greater risk to your health than being obese. And while exercise may not be the best method of losing weight, being active has been shown to increase the likelihood of *maintaining* any weight loss achieved. It also improves so many other factors (sleep, energy, and mood) that it may help to improve our ability to make better dietary decisions as a result. I spend considerably more time discussing exercise benefits and goals in the next chapter. The bottom line is that, when it comes to weight loss and weight maintenance, you will have a much higher chance of success by focusing on your diet. *You cannot outrun your fork.*

Food as Reward

Presently, the world is set up such that high-caloric junk foods are used as a constant and expected reward for the most minimal and meaningless activities. Pizza days are held at school on a regular basis. Desserts are standard following most meals. Treats are provided at school and the office for holidays and birthdays. Fundraisers typically involve the sale of candies and chocolate bars. Thank you treats tend to be food-related and are apt to be cookies, cakes, doughnuts, or muffins, rather than fruit or vegetable trays.

This increased prevalence of junk food used as incentives and rewards creates a perverse relationship with food and an expectation of junk. This is unfortunately not likely to change in and of itself anytime soon, so it is something of which to be aware.

Given that backdrop, it is no wonder that making meaningful dietary choices resulting in long-lasting weight loss is hard. There is no easy answer and no quick fix. But there are changes that can be made and it is possible to successfully eat better—with or without weight loss. In order to succeed, you need to remember *why* you are doing this. Why do you want to be healthier? Why do you want to eat better and smarter? Why do you want to try to lose weight?

To that end, think about your ignition statement from the previous chapter, "Change" (page 40) to ensure that your inspiration is front and center. *Why do you deserve to make the best dietary choices for your body each and every day? Because...*

Five Dietary Principles

The next step is to go over some guiding principles that provide a framework for you to view your dietary choices and then make concrete plans to improve them. These values and beliefs help keep your focus on the practical solutions required to make real change.

1. Calories Matter

If you look at your diet and what you put into your body as a currency, then you have to know what your budget is. Similar to finances, you can't do that without knowing your income and expenses. Calories are simply a tool to measure the amount of energy a food contains and how much energy a particular activity burns. Is it perfect? No. Are all the calories the same? Probably not. But is there a better way to traverse the food landscape? Nope.

Given that you are using calories as the means of keeping track of what goes in and out of your body, why do we focus predominantly on the calories you ingest and not equally on what you burn?

When you look at the calories that you take in, it is *only* from the food and drink you consume; you aren't producing any calories from the sun or by wearing special shoes. In contrast, you burn calories in *multiple* ways, the largest portion being your basal metabolic rate (BMR). Your BMR is the energy used to run your body at rest, accounting for 60 to 80 percent of the energy you use. Another 10 percent is burned just digesting and processing the food you eat. So, looking at the math, that only leaves 10 to 30 percent left to be burned through exercise (dedicated physical activity) and normal movement (walking to the bathroom, doing chores, etc.).

Another problem is that, if and when you do exercise, you tend to justify sitting more, doing less normal activity, and maybe eating a few extra calories. As a result, your total calories burned usually stays the same, or those additional calories you eat quickly offsets the extra calories burned. That does not negate all of the other many benefits exercise provides; it's just worth keeping in mind as part of the overall calculation.

Dr. Mark Haub, a nutrition professor at Kansas State University, personally demonstrated that the quantity of calories you ingest may well be more important than the quality. In 2010, Dr. Haub was able to lose twenty-seven pounds over two months by eating fewer calories than he burned, even though the food he ate consisted solely of Twinkies, Doritos, Oreos, and other junk foods. This is obviously not a recommended diet but is an example of how the tracking of calories may trump the diet itself.

In fact, the reason that any trendy diet works is that it limits the number of calories consumed. A diet that incorporates shakes as meal replacements is decreasing your caloric intake by controlling the number of calories in the shake. A low-carb diet or high-protein diet tends to cause people to feel fuller (since proteins are more filling than carbs), thus resulting in fewer calories overall. A diet that vilifies any particular food group limits calories by restricting the choices to be made. Intermittent fasting decreases total calories ingested by limiting the hours that you can eat. Weight Watchers or other points-based systems use those points instead of calories for the same purpose of tracking how much you eat.

The bottom line is that your first step in gaining control of your diet is becoming aware of the number of calories in the food you eat and how many calories are required to maintain your body weight. Use an online calorie calculator to determine your daily caloric requirements based on weight, height, and activity levels. Then eat 500 calories fewer than that to aim for a weight loss rate of approximately one pound per week. Granted, this balance will change as you lose weight and reach a new plateau so, as you progress, you will need to redo the calculation periodically.

2. Suffering Is to Be Avoided

The next guiding principle to keep in mind is that you are not wired to suffer for long periods of time. You can endure things for a while, but it is not sustainable as a long-term weight-loss plan. Millions of people are able to tolerate all manner of difficult diets and lose weight *temporarily* by shear willpower. I am always amazed and impressed by the strength it must take to endure some of these diets for even a few weeks.

However, the inevitable reality is that if you are not able to feel happy on a diet and to sustain the changes continually, then the weight lost will return and often even more than that. This is the unfortunate fact of most diets and the reason for the yo-yo dieting phenomenon.

The good news is that suffering need not be a requirement of a diet, and it actually *has* to be absent in order for an enduring dietary change to stick. The result is that the pounds will come off at a slower rate, but slow and steady is definitely preferred for successful long-term weight loss.

3. Your Best Weight Is Good Enough

Dr. Freedhoff describes something called your "best weight" in his book *The Diet Fix*, my go-to diet resource recommendation. This is the weight you achieve while living the healthiest life you *enjoy*, in keeping with our "no suffering" policy, which makes it much more doable.

In Tal Ben-Shahar's *Happier*, he describes why he titled his book as he did: it is possible for all of us to work toward being *happier*, but if our goal is being *happy*, then that's a much more nebulous and difficult thing to achieve. Similarly, we can all find ways to be healthier, thinner, or fitter and succeed in that without having the immense pressure of reaching an ultimate goal of being "healthy," "thin," or "fit," whatever those terms actually mean. Just focus on the "-er" and be content with that.

4. Hunger Is Your Enemy

Have you ever gone grocery shopping while hungry? How about hitting the drive-through after a long and busy day at work? How healthy and thoughtful were your choices? I don't know about you, but in those scenarios, I tend to buy more junk food, upsize the combo, or generally make the worst decisions regarding diet.

Eating only when you are hungry may seem like a reasonable solution to eating less, but we tend to not make the best choices in that state. If you plan ahead and schedule your snacks and meals, you can better manage your food decisions, ensure you are getting the nutrients you need, and avoid the suffering of true hunger.

Evolutionarily speaking, hunger is one of the most powerful drives we have; ignore it at your peril. If you are regularly hungry on your diet, then it will not be sustainable and your body will fight against you. The goal is to eat enough calories to lose weight without feeling hungry all day. This is possible and doable, provided you plan for it and expect slow and steady progress toward your desired objective.

5. There Are *No* Forbidden Foods

Life is too precious to ban chocolate and cake and those amazing pastries available at your local bakery. Food serves so many purposes in society—as a means of celebration, grief, socializing, and pleasure. You would be doing yourself a disservice if you didn't allow yourself the opportunity to take part in those offerings.

However, you need to understand that those delectable treats are just that: treats. If you have a high-calorie dessert daily or a cookie with every coffee break, they are no longer special. Dr. Freedhoff suggests you ask two simple questions about any type of food that is not a necessary part of your diet but is something that you enjoy:

1. Is it worth the calories?
2. What is the smallest amount I need to be happy?

There are no right or wrong answers to these questions; it is a value judgment we each need to make. But I'm sure you've had the experience of eating some sort of junk food, candy bar, or dessert and not even enjoying it. Or, upon learning the calorie content of what you just ate, you realize what you could have had instead for the same amount. "I could have had two chocolate bars instead of that mediocre banana walnut bread?"

Similarly, we've all had the sensation of that first incredible bite of a dessert, but then, by the end, it's too sweet and too much. Yet many of us still finish it. Aim to have the smallest amount you need to feel you've had enough—whether that's chocolate, ice cream, chips, soda, or whatever is your treat.

There is room for anything if you need it to be happy, but ask those two key questions before mindlessly eating it. That way, you can enjoy them fully, consciously, and without the guilt.

Seven Key Actions

Now that we've reviewed the challenges in changing how we eat and the main principles guiding how we think about it, it is time to focus on some specific behaviors to help make changes.

1. Keep a Food Diary

The reality is that keeping account of what you eat, when you eat, and the caloric cost of the foods you eat is necessary for dietary change. As I said earlier, it would be like trying to keep a balanced financial budget but not keeping track of income and expenditures—it's impossible. Now it may seem like a lot of work initially but, with time and the use of various tools, it can be done very quickly and efficiently.

It also may not seem fair that you have to do this seemingly cumbersome activity when others don't, but the reality is that some people are able to remain slim without diarizing because of their genetics, upbringing, emotional state, palate, intense physical activity levels, and who knows what else. That is not our concern; what we do know is that if people desire to lose weight and change how they eat, keeping a food diary *doubles* the amount of weight they lose. The more detailed the diary, the more weight is lost!

The main purpose of a food diary is information: it is used to make better decisions in the future, not to judge past choices. One big lesson that is learned quickly when keeping track of calories is appropriate portion size—and this alone can lead to significant insight in future food choices. Today it is easier than ever to keep track of caloric intake and increase your chances of success. Food diaries are available in any number of formats: a written journal, free online service, or smartphone application. Just remember to first determine your daily caloric needs as a means of providing context to your choices.

2. Cook More and Eat Out Less

As soon as you leave home and eat at a restaurant, or choose to eat prepared foods, you are likely to dramatically overshoot your caloric goals. Cooking and eating at home is one of the best things you can do to control your dietary choices and eat better. It need not be complicated; find a few recipes you enjoy and take the time to learn a new one every few weeks to expand your repertoire, confidence, and skills. You can also try cooking with friends to share recipes, techniques, skills—and the food.

3. Eat Less Processed Food

You may have noticed that I have not written much about which foods are the best to eat. I believe that people all have their own palates, choices, and biases. Even if there was ample evidence that the low-carb diet is the best diet ever (there isn't—but it doesn't seem to be bad either), it is unlikely pasta, rice, or bread will disappear given their historical, ethnic, and cultural prominence in many diets—and that's okay.

The main parameter to focus on is buying and eating food made from simple and basic ingredients. This means purchasing and eating real food that is predominantly located around the periphery of a grocery store—fresh (or frozen) fruits and vegetables, meat and fish, whole grains, nuts, legumes, and dairy—and avoiding the processed stuff in boxes in the middle aisles. Now this doesn't mean you can't and shouldn't buy processed food at all; there's no judgment here. Simply try to minimize it as best you can and focus on those same two questions regarding treats: is it worth it, and what is the least amount of it you can have to be happy?

For further details on what specific foods to eat and in what proportions, the Harvard Healthy Eating Plate and Healthy Eating Pyramid offer a great visual and reference resource. They recommend that half your plate be made up of vegetables and fruit (potatoes don't count), a quarter to be whole grains, and the remaining quarter to consist of a protein source (ideally limiting red and processed meat). Plant oils should also be included in moderation, and they advise limiting milk/dairy to only one or two servings per day.

If you want specific support with your eating, I highly encourage you to consult a registered dietitian (RD). These individuals are part of a regulated profession and have been trained via a four-year university program along with internships and regular continuing education. While some RDs (like in any profession) may give bad advice not grounded in science, the vast majority are reliable given their standardized education. They are much more reliable than a "nutritionist," as this designation is not regulated and can be obtained via an unaccredited online course or simply by declaring yourself one.

A brief aside about organic and non-GMO foods: the evidence is not there to support the claim that eating these foods is healthier than other foods. There are a lot of reasons people choose these items—moral, environmental, personal, philosophical—and I don't want to get into the specifics around those reasons, but these foods don't seem to directly correlate with improved health. It is far more important to eat more fruits and vegetables, period, than it is to eat organic.

My concern is that people may overspend for these specific items, eat fewer fruits and vegetables as a result of the cost, or feel that they can't afford healthy food due to the markup. I also would hope that people don't purchase boxed foods labeled organic over nonorganic, for example, thinking they're healthy when they are still processed foods high in calories. Eating simple whole foods is better than eating processed foods, even if the box proclaims it is organic. I would consider eating organic as a form of "supplement" and would recommend using the same process of consideration I outline in chapter 10.

Whatever avenue you wish to pursue in eating healthier, no simpler motto can be found than author Michael Pollan's oft-quoted line from *In Defense of Food*: "Eat food. Not too much. Mostly plants."

4. Look at Nutritional Labels

In making smart food choices and avoiding processed foods, it is a good idea to become comfortable using the information on nutritional labels to guide your decisions.

The first line to look at is the *total calories per serving*. This helps you determine how much the food "costs" in a caloric sense. But be certain to also look at the *serving size*. It is easy to get confused. The label on a bag of chips or chocolates states a certain number of calories, but you may not have realized the bag (which you just ate the entire contents of) contained four servings, not one.

Next, it is worth noting the amount of *protein*, as eating adequate amounts of protein helps stave off hunger. Dietitians recommend at least 0.8 grams of protein daily for every kilogram of weight, while Dr. Freedhoff suggests aiming for more with at least 20 grams of protein with each meal and 10 grams for each snack.

Take a look at the amount of *sugar* (per serving) on the label as well, since we can all consume less sugar overall. If you are looking at ingredient lists, understand that many different names can be given to items used to sweeten foods (sugar, cane sugar, brown sugar, honey, fruit juice concentrate, high fructose corn syrup) but they are all equivalent to sugar and should be minimized. Also be aware that many foods advertised as "low fat" will have added sugars to boost flavor—there's always a trade-off.

In fact, another trick is to ignore *all* front-of-package health claims (low fat, low cholesterol, high fiber, rich in antioxidants) and focus on the basic information on the nutrition label (as mentioned above) as well as the ingredient list, which should be short and understandable. Consider the claims on the front to be advertisements.

Keep these simple tips in mind and you should be better able to navigate the complexities of food labeling when selecting food at the grocery store.

5. Minimize Liquid Calories

When you drink your calories, they do not make you feel fuller; they just add to your daily intake. For example, if you were to drink a 200-calorie beverage with your meal instead of water, you will not typically eat 200 calories less as a result. You've just added extra calories to your meal. Eliminating or decreasing these calories is often the simplest and easiest way to decrease your daily caloric intake. Also consider your alcohol intake; beyond its calories, alcohol can reduce willpower and can cause one to eat more as well.

Juice, soda, alcohol, and high-calorie caffeinated beverages are extremely common and unnecessary sources of calories that can add up quickly. It is shocking how many calories are in some of the fancy caffeinated beverages—a tall caramel Frappuccino, even with 2 percent milk and no whipped cream, comes in at more than 200 calories; that's more than a glazed doughnut!

CALORIES IN ALCOHOL

Type	Serving Size	Approximate Calories
Red or white wine	5 oz	120
Most beer	12 oz	150
Most spirits (no mix)	1.5 oz	100
Most liqueurs	1 oz	100

The best bet is to limit your beverages to just water, coffee, and tea (with no sugar and low or nonfat milk, if any). Even milk should be considered with caution, as it can often be a source of significant extra calories; again, try to limit milk and dairy products to one or two daily servings only. If you do need to have a sweetened beverage, then using artificial sweeteners is a valid and safe alternative, but be aware that there is some weak evidence that their use makes people crave other sweetened foods.

A small aside about fruit juice—it is simply sugar and water with a different name than soda but similar caloric counts. Any nutrient benefit from fruit juice is lost in the processing and is definitely not the same as eating a piece of fruit. Treat juice and other sources of liquid calories as an indulgence like any other: be sure it's worth it and have the smallest amount you need.

Alcohol: Low-Risk Drinking Guidelines

Alcohol is an interesting and confusing substance in that it is obviously associated with significant health issues—addiction, liver disease, increased cancer risk, unplanned pregnancies, violence, poor decision-making, accidents—but it is also suggested to be beneficial for heart health. And, of course, it doesn't seem like alcohol will be leaving our society anytime soon.

Given that, what are the guidelines for drinking alcohol in a healthy and low-risk manner? Both the Canadian Centre on Substance Abuse and Addiction and the American Centers for Disease Control and Prevention have provided some rules to consider.

Don't drink alcohol at all if:

- You don't already drink and don't wish to start. There is not enough evidence to recommend drinking solely as a preventive strategy.
- You are or may be pregnant.
- You are under the legal drinking age.
- You are a recovering alcoholic or someone unable to control how much you drink.
- You are doing something that requires skill, coordination, and alertness—like driving a car.
- You are on medication or have a medical condition which may be affected by alcohol.

Low-risk drinking guidelines:

- Women should limit themselves to *no more* than ten drinks/ week with *no more* than two drinks a day.
- Men should limit themselves to *no more* than fifteen drinks/ week with *no more* than three drinks a day.
- A drink is defined as 12 oz of 5 percent beer/cider/cooler, 5 oz of 12 percent wine, or 1.5 oz of 40 percent hard liquor.
- Plan on having nondrinking days regularly to reduce the risk of developing a habit.

- Drink slowly with no more than two drinks within three hours.

- Eat before and while you drink.

- Have one nonalcoholic beverage for each alcoholic one.

- Stick to the limits you set for yourself and be aware of any personal reasons (health, age, experience, body weight) that may warrant lowering them.

- For celebrations or special occasions, be sure to limit yourself to *no more* than three drinks (for women) or four drinks (for men), keeping the above guidelines in mind.

6. Eat at Regular Intervals

In order to avoid hunger, it is important to plan ahead and eat regularly. This typically requires eating three meals and three snacks per day. Aim to eat every two to three hours—even if you're not hungry. Remember, hunger is a form of suffering that you are trying to avoid and you tend to make your worst dietary decisions when feeling it.

You want to plan such that each snack and meal has sufficient calories to ensure it lasts to the next one. This is individualized so some people may be able to stave off hunger with only three meals while others need more of a "grazing" approach. The goal is to find an eating pattern that suits you for the long term so your priority is to ensure you don't feel hungry and are happy with your approach.

Protein tends to be more filling than carbohydrates, so incorporating enough protein into your meals helps you feel more satisfied. I find that most people have a reasonable sense of how to incorporate protein into their meals but can struggle when considering snack options. The majority of snacks we resort to are carbohydrate-heavy—chips, granola bars, and crackers, for example. It is worth figuring out some acceptable protein-rich snacks you enjoy and have them on hand for a quick, healthy choice. Some ideas include almonds or other nuts, hummus and pita, cheese with or without crackers, a peanut butter sandwich, or boiled eggs.

A typical snack size for the average male should be at least 150 calories; for a meal, at least 400 calories. For the average female, the minimum snack size should be 100 calories; for a meal, at least 300 calories. You may need to adjust these amounts as required in order to meet daily caloric targets and to avoid hunger.

7. Eat Breakfast

In keeping with the plan of eating regularly and consistently, studies suggest that eating breakfast is a healthy choice to help lose and maintain body weight. The National Weight Control Registry, a group which follows and tracks thousands of people in the United States who have succeeded in losing weight (the average is sixty-seven pounds kept off for 5.5 years), found that 78 percent report they eat breakfast daily.

Eating breakfast seems be a factor that favors weight loss, so most professionals recommend it, although it is a weaker recommendation. It may be difficult initially, since those who do not tend to eat breakfast get their full caloric intake in the latter half of the day and don't feel hungry in the morning. Once that adjustment is made, however, the day can flow more smoothly with the first meal setting the pace.

Summary

Eating is one of the great pleasures of life, but it can also be a source of great suffering. It is intimidating and challenging to face this landscape of easily accessible, high-caloric, and low-quality food. Understandably, it can be exhausting to resist the temptations and not feel deprived, but with practical strategies in place, it can be done.

The general framework for eating well may require you to keep track of calories but should not cause you to suffer or feel hungry. You need to allow yourself the joy of having your favorite foods but eat them mindfully and be aware of their caloric costs. And most importantly, you need to aim for eating better, as a healthy diet is clearly an important foundation to healthy living—with or without weight loss.

Within that framework, you can then focus on specific actions to improve your diet: keeping a food diary, cooking more, shopping mindfully, minimizing liquid calories, and eating regularly, including breakfast. These behaviors are conducive to setting SMART goals and thus can be measured and monitored on your journey to eating better and losing weight, if desired. There are lots of potential ways to target your diet and it is up to you to decide which concrete choices make the best sense for your life.

A saying I first heard in the surgical world, but which was originally said by Voltaire and is widely applicable, is that "perfect is the enemy of good." This applies to diet as well. You don't need to be perfect: you just need to be better. Focus on creating the absolute healthiest diet and life you can *enjoy*, and find contentment and satisfaction in that.

4

Move

"To enjoy the glow of good health, you must exercise."
Gene Tunney

EXERCISE IS KNOWN to be a key requirement to healthy living but unfortunately, for many of us, it seems like a grueling means of torture that must be endured. Humans are not good at suffering for long periods of time, and so we shouldn't be surprised we can't sustain an activity that we view so negatively. To that end, I would alter nineteenth-century American boxer Gene Tunney's quote and say that we must *enjoy* exercise to enjoy good health.

When I see patients who are healthy and fit, inevitably a big component of that is regular physical activity, whether it's as involved as running marathons or simply making a daily walk a priority. Thankfully, there is no shortage of different forms of activity and, with just a little bit of effort, I'm certain you can find something that brings you joy.

For many people, finding time and energy for exercise can be challenging. But exercise may well be the best thing you can do for your health; without a doubt, it's worth it—its benefits cannot be matched. If you want to live your best life, you need to make exercise a priority, not an afterthought. It needs to be planned, scheduled, and emphasized. Increased physical activity can improve your mood, energy, and sleep, and it decreases your risk of many health issues. It is even associated with increasing the joy in your life. Exercising regularly is something I do as part of my goal to be healthy but also as part of my goal to be happy.

Regrettably, the majority of people have not found their reasons and their own best way to work out and, as a result, simply do not exercise. In 2008, the American Centers for Disease Control and Prevention found that 25 percent of people surveyed had not done any physical activity in the past month, and less than half had achieved the target of thirty minutes of activity five times a week. In Canada, it was worse, with less than a third having reached the targets for physical activity.

Increasing the number of people moving from a sedentary and inactive lifestyle to a more active one is one of the best interventions we could make to improve the overall wellness of our population. But again, we need to be specific in terms of the goals we set and why. The results that people expect from exercise may differ greatly from the impressive benefits they are actually receiving.

Patients often acknowledge they would like to lose some weight and immediately discuss their plan to become more active to shed the pounds. As mentioned in the "Eat" chapter, exercise does not seem to be the most effective way to lose weight. It is possible to lose pounds with exercise—if you dramatically increase your level of activity and consciously focus on not increasing your caloric intake—but your chances of success are much higher if you focus on diet.

If, as a result of increasing your physical activity, you are expecting to lose large amounts of weight, develop a six-pack, and/or have a body like your favorite actor's, then you are likely to be disappointed. Instead, you have to focus on how exercise can positively affect your important health factors and lead to *decreased burden of illness* and *increased enjoyment of life*. These are far more valuable and more enduring than the superficial and temporary benefits of looking good for your wedding or beach holiday. Plus, they are more sustainable and realistic.

If you are disenchanted or saddened by the truth that exercising alone is not likely to get you ripped or on the cover of a magazine, I hope to encourage you by the sheer magnitude of other meaningful benefits that exercise provides. The actual gains you receive from improving your physical activity levels are much more impressive, much broader in scope, and much more consequential than any superficial change could ever be. Truly, the tangible benefits of even the smallest increases in physical activity are incredible.

Benefits of Increased Movement

The benefits of increased activity are widespread, improving almost all aspects of health. This is why exercise is often called the *one best thing you can do for your health*. A great video that summarizes this information is Dr. Mike Evans's "23 and ½ Hours," which has been viewed more than eight million times. This short and entertaining video looks at why exercising for just thirty minutes a day is the single best intervention you can do for your overall wellness.

Here are some of the many returns you can get with your investment of a little bit of time and energy:

- decreased risk of death
- decreased risk of dementia

- decreased risk of developing type 2 diabetes
- decreased risk of heart attack and stroke
- decreased risk of osteoarthritis
- decreased risk of colon cancer
- decreased risk of breast cancer
- decreased risk of falls and hip fractures
- decreased levels of pain
- decreased risk of anxiety
- increased energy
- increased quality of life
- improved quality of sleep
- improved maintenance of weight

I could have spent a lot of time listing study results, going over all the evidence that supports the above statements, and quantifying them in great detail; however, this information is rarely helpful in motivating people to make this behavioral change. (Although I have listed references at the end of the book for those interested.) With such information, I am only speaking to your brain and not to your heart. You need to find your own deep reasons to *feel the need to change* and start moving.

So, I will ask you again to think of your personal ignition statement from "Change"—that one reminder that drives you to do and be your best.

Why do you deserve to make the effort, find the time, and discover the energy to increase your level of physical activity each and every day? Because...

(This is not a trick question; the answer should be the same as your original ignition statement.)

Activity vs. Exercise

When looking to increase your levels of activity, it is worth distinguishing between exercise and activity—and acknowledging the value of both. *Physical activity* is defined as any actions or movements of the body that use energy beyond that which is used by the body at rest. Activity includes daily and routine tasks such as walking to or around at work, taking the stairs, folding laundry, cooking, doing dishes, gardening, and yard work.

Exercise is a subtype of physical activity that is planned, structured, and repetitive with a goal to improve physical fitness on some level.

Physical fitness is defined by the *New World Encyclopedia* as "the body's ability to function effectively and efficiently in work and leisure activities, not only at a set point in time but at various ages and stages within a person's life cycle." This ability can be measured to some degree in terms of aerobic capacity (e.g., walking, running, cycling), muscular strength (e.g., amount of weight one can lift), muscular endurance (e.g., number of push-ups possible), flexibility (e.g., touching toes), and body composition (e.g., body fat percentage).

For the purposes of this book, I will use the term *physical activity* to refer solely to those activities done in the course of normal day-to-day exertion and *exercise* as a separate structured action. Both are important and crucial to health, weight maintenance, and physical fitness.

Make Your Day Harder

Dr. Mike Evans has created a movement (and another great video) to motivate all of us to increase the amount of activity in our regular day: Make Your Day Harder. We spend the vast majority of our time sitting, so much so that sitting is now considered a major risk factor for illness and disease. Studies have shown that people who are more sedentary die sooner—regardless of cause—than those who are less so. Sitting has also been shown to be associated with increased risk of heart disease, diabetes, cancer, and hospitalizations. Not to state that these conditions are *caused* by sitting, as being inactive can also be a *result* of other health issues; however, there really is no doubt that sitting for long periods is not good for you, and taking time to get up and move is of great benefit.

Our days have also gotten much easier as a result of technology and our modern lifestyles. We tend to drive everywhere, and our work and leisure activities have become much more sedentary. Few of us walk to work anymore, but one study out of Japan showed that those who did so had better health outcomes than those who didn't, and the farther the walk, the bigger the difference.

We also use computers and screens for the majority of our jobs with less intrinsic activity at work; we rarely even have to get up to make copies or go to the printer anymore. And our recreational activities also tend to be focused on screens, with television, Netflix, and internet taking up the majority of our evening hours. In a Nielsen Total Audience Report, it was found that the average adult was on a screen of some sort for ten hours and thirty-nine minutes each day.

Clearly, we can afford to make our days a bit harder, and it all adds up. As a family physician, I am fortunate to have the opportunity to walk and move around throughout the course of my regular workday. A colleague of mine, a fellow family physician, retrained to be a radiologist, a doctor who reads X-rays full-time. He is an incredibly fit guy who watches what he eats and exercises regularly. He soon realized that this change in career, which had him sitting at a workstation reading images for hours at a time, was causing him to gain weight. There was no other change in his diet or exercise routine, other than the fact that his regular workday got easier with more sitting time. Even small changes in activity can have significant impact.

Standing more and sitting less is one useful way to make your day harder, but it is too nonspecific for my liking. I want to provide you with concrete ways to make positive changes in your health. Here is a list of ideas that you could incorporate to increase the degree of difficulty of your average day.

Ideas to Make Your Day Harder

1. Park farther away from your destination to allow you to walk a bit more.

2. Take the stairs instead of the elevator or escalator.

3. Stand up whenever you are on the phone.

4. Replace your coffee break with a quick walk.

5. Rather than wheeling your chair around your office, stand up and walk to get what you need.

6. Walk to your colleague's office to ask them a question rather than calling or emailing them.

7. Set a reminder to stand for five minutes out of every hour.

8. Look at incorporating a sit-to-stand workstation in your office.

9. Go for a brisk walk at lunch.

10. Do housework or yard work with a little extra effort and be happy for the opportunity to work harder.

11. Use a pedometer or Fitbit and measure your daily steps. Aim for 10,000 per day. (Most of us require a dedicated walk or run to reach that goal.)

12. Walk on the treadmill while watching your favorite show or walk outside while listening to your favorite podcast.

13. Walk or cycle to work when able.

14. If taking public transit to work, get off a stop or two early and walk the rest of the way.

15. Play with your kids—kick the soccer ball, throw a ball around, roughhouse, explore.

16. Get a dog and appreciate the regular walking companion and motivator.

17. Wash and wax your car by hand rather than using an automatic carwash.

18. Have sex more often. (No one said adding more activity to your day couldn't be enjoyable!)

19. At work, use the washroom farthest away from your workstation.

20. While watching television, exercise (try some push-ups or plank) or stretch during commercials.

Sweat, Smile, Repeat

As stated earlier, exercise is physical activity that is planned, structured, and repetitive with a goal to improve physical fitness and provide enjoyment. Incorporating purposeful exercise in addition to physical activity is strongly recommended to add years to your life. The general recommendation for adults is to get a minimum of *150 minutes of moderately vigorous exercise each week.* "Moderately vigorous" can be easily thought of as activity that simply makes you sweat. That recommendation divides neatly to thirty minutes five times a week, but it should be noted that this is considered a minimum recommendation; there is no good evidence to suggest there's an upper limit to the benefits of exercise.

How Much Exercise Is Needed?

Alex Hutchinson, PhD, makes a lot of excellent points in his science-based book on fitness, *Which Comes First, Cardio or Weights?* One in particular is as follows:

> "Decades of research have made two things crystal clear:
>
> 1. Every bit of exercise helps, even in scraps as short as ten minutes.
> 2. More is almost always better.
>
> The challenge is conveying the second message without discouraging the people who are still struggling with the first."

I see this challenge all the time in my medical practice. Notes come back from cardiologists or other specialists stating that they recommended to the patient that they reduce their cardiovascular risk by increasing their physical activity to the recommended 150 minutes/week. I wonder how successful they honestly think that advice will be. Just do it? That advice is probably about as useful as the age-old "eat less, exercise more" recommendation—accurate but not that helpful.

Every bit of exercise helps your health, so add some to your day or week in any way you can. Setting unrealistic goals can be discouraging and that is one thing we need to avoid. The goal is to encourage you to move from an inactive, sedentary life to a more active one; even just starting to walk a few minutes a day may be a reasonable and terrific place to start on your path to wellness. That decision deserves celebration and support. But you should always try to add more exercise until you are living the most active life you can enjoy.

Now let's look at some specific actions to help you on that path.

The Best Exercise

There are so many types of exercise and I'm often asked if one specific activity is better than any other in terms of fitness. The answer to that is fairly simple. Yes, there is one exercise that is better than the rest: *the one you will actually do.*

Just as with diet, where suffering is not sustainable and the goal is to find the healthiest diet you can enjoy, the goal with exercise is to find the activity that you enjoy enough that it becomes a part of your regular life. It really doesn't matter what you choose as long you can see yourself continuing it for the long term. Here are some possibilities:

- walking
- running
- skiing—cross-country or downhill
- snowshoeing
- dancing
- team sports—e.g., basketball, hockey, soccer, volleyball
- weight lifting
- yoga
- skating
- rollerblading
- rock climbing or bouldering
- swimming
- aerobics, spin classes, or any other group exercise class
- martial arts

- hiking
- exercise machines, like a treadmill or elliptical
- mountain biking or road cycling
- rowing
- boot camps
- tennis or other racquet sports

All of these are excellent choices to add exercise and enjoyment to your life. I'm sure there are many others that you could think of that would be equally appropriate. Again, the biggest and most important factor is finding something that you enjoy and will find time to do.

Progress Is Key

An important feature of any successful exercise program is seeing progress. This helps move you to higher and higher states of fitness, as your body gets used to your initial workout routine and the previously "moderately vigorous" exercise becomes easier. In order to see this change occur in yourself, you will need to create some specific short- and long-term goals and measure your outcomes.

Use the same SMART goals system we discussed in "Change" —successful goals are *specific, measurable, attainable, relevant,* and *time specific*. In addition to that acronym, we can add FITT to the list, which further details the "specific" of SMART.

Frequency—the number of times per week you plan on doing the activity.

Intensity—could refer to the pace of the treadmill or elliptical machine, the amount of weight lifted, the number of push-ups, or the "light" versus "moderate" pace of your walk.

Type—the specific type of exercise you will be doing (e.g., attending a yoga class, going for a walk, doing a spin class).

Time—the specific duration of each exercise session—ten, twenty, or thirty minutes, for example. (This is distinct from the "time" in SMART, which refers to how long you plan on doing this goal—two, four, or six weeks, for example.)

You could set a goal of walking at a moderate pace for fifteen minutes and do that three times per week. Let's look at that goal in more detail in regards to FITT and SMART.

- *Specific:* By their nature, FITT goals offer an outline to create specific exercise goals, but more specificity always helps. In addition to the FITT features—frequency (three times/week), intensity (moderately paced), type (walking), and time (fifteen minutes)—you could add additional information such as which days you will walk, at what time of day, and maybe even the route.

- *Measurable:* Exercise goals are easily measurable—it is only a matter of recording in a book, journal, calendar, or smartphone app the days the workout was done.

- *Attainable:* You need to be confident you can achieve your exercise goals, so that you can build from success. You should feel at least 80 percent confident that you can walk for fifteen minutes three times a week; if not, adjust your target.

- *Relevant:* The goal of walking more is in keeping with your overall desire of being healthier. It should also be in keeping with your ignition statement and relate back to the ultimate reason of why you want to be well.

- *Time-limited:* You should set a period of time to complete this particular goal before reassessing and reevaluating. Perhaps it's reasonable to try this plan for four weeks before seeing if you need to make it harder (or easier) in some way.

Is Walking Enough?

Many people wonder if going for a daily walk is enough activity to see significant benefits. If that is the only activity you are able to do and you do it consistently, you will see improvements in many areas of your health compared to doing nothing. In my practice, I have numerous elderly patients who maintain good health and include a regular walk as their main form of exercise. All exercise is beneficial, but the more you do, the better the benefits. The evidence is more supportive for those who are "briskly" walking: swinging your arms forcefully, striding purposefully, and being able to speak but needing pauses to catch your breath.

If you are currently inactive and looking for a place to start, walking is absolutely a great place to do so. It requires no fancy equipment, is free, and only requires the time to put on your shoes and walk out the door. Even Hippocrates, the ancient Greek founder of medicine, considered that "walking is [our] best medicine."

As you feel able, you can push yourself slowly and steadily to increased duration, frequency, and intensity. Who knows—maybe as you progress, you will be able to start moving toward running or other exercises. But the greatest gains for the health of the individual, and the public in general, are seen when people change from being sedentary and inactive to becoming active. So if you feel like walking is the limit to what you can reasonably add to your day, that's okay—the idea is to live the healthiest life you can enjoy, and walking can certainly be a great part of that.

Running

If you want to progress further and continue to push yourself, running would be the next logical step. Running is a harder activity and burns significantly more calories than walking—how much more is up for debate but probably in the range of 1.5 to 2.5 times as many. More important than the increased calories burned, however, is your body's increased effort and thus the increased benefits your body will gain. This is due to the increased pace as well as the fact that, when running, with each stride you are pushing your body into the air (albeit only slightly and for a moment), which takes a bit more force.

There are many running programs and groups to join in most towns and cities to help people slowly advance to their first run, and I'm always impressed by how supportive and positive the running community is. Group dynamics are a powerful way to keep motivated, and I would highly recommend using that to your advantage.

Alternatively, you can look at structured programs to get started running on your own. England's National Health Service has a very simple Couch to 5K program which outlines a progressive schedule to help people gradually be able to run five kilometers without stopping. Dr. James Beckerman, a cardiologist, has written a very practical book called *Heart to Start* to likewise help get people moving and increase their fitness. I heard Dr. Beckerman speak at a conference a few years ago and was impressed with his passion for preventive medicine and the value of exercise. He is truly a believer in the benefits of getting the least active of us moving, demonstrated by his Heart to Start program.

Strength vs. Cardio

I have always enjoyed strength training (lifting weights, yoga, body-weight exercises), often more so than aerobic activities (running, cycling), although that is changing as the years go on. There are numerous benefits to resistance training, which you will not get from doing strictly aerobic activities. Similarly, there are benefits from cardio activities that you don't get from weight training. Ideally, you can find ways to eventually incorporate both into your weekly routine.

The typical debate around strength training versus cardio concerns which is better for weight loss. We have already established that while exercise has an incredible number of benefits, weight loss should not be a primary one. Taking that out of the equation, we find that strength training does wonders to maintain muscle mass and bone mass, thus reducing the risk of falls and fractures. If done at a good pace and intensity, strength training qualifies as part of your 150 minutes of vigorous physical activity per week.

The key to a good strength-training program is slow and steady progression, so you are always pushing your body to work harder. Most simply, this involves a gradual increase in the amount of weight lifted or an increase in the number of repetitions done—being sure to maintain good form. A personal trainer may help ensure you are doing the activity properly. Please be cautious in selecting a trainer and find one with good accreditation (American College of Sports Medicine [ACSM] and National Strength and Conditioning Association [NSCA] are well-respected organizations but are still no guarantee). You also want someone with a good reputation, so ask people you trust for a recommendation. Also keep in mind that you want someone who will focus on what *your* goals are, teach you how to do the exercises properly, and then allow you to graduate, so you can continue progressing on your own without the ongoing cost associated with having a personal trainer (unless you find that a valuable and enjoyable motivation tool).

Weight training provides clear positive feedback in regards to how much strength you have gained, which can be motivating. Also, people who are overweight tend to have quite good strength, so it can be a form of exercise that helps build confidence. In addition, the pace of the workout allows for some intense exertion followed by periods of rest, which can be more accommodating than the ongoing exertion typically expected with cardio activities.

Some very simple and effective routines involve using your body weight and focusing on functional movements. They require very little equipment and can often be easily done at home. Yoga classes, the use of resistance bands, or TRX suspension training are also very effective strength training workouts. I've done a number of programs like that and they were surprisingly as challenging, if not more so, than many weight routines I've done.

One other workout I have done periodically is the 100 push-up, twenty pull-up, and 100 squat challenges. These workouts are straightforward, structured, and advance you slowly up to the target. There is a freedom in not having to think about what the next routine will be as you just do the prescribed numbers of repetitions and sets. These workouts tend to be three times a week and take about twenty to thirty minutes to do. But even if you don't achieve the ultimate target of 100 push-ups or twenty pull-ups (which can be pretty daunting), you will still experience significant strength gains as you progress as far as you can.

If you are looking for a more typical weight lifting workout, an excellent place to start is the StrongLifts 5x5 routine, which is based on the recommendations from Mark Rippetoe's classic workout book *Starting Strength*. It consists of two workouts that alternate three days a week. The exercises include the basic barbell exercises of the squat, bench press, overhead press, deadlift, and barbell row. These movements target multiple muscles and thus are all that is needed to get a full body workout. After finding an appropriate starting weight to lift in each exercise (with this workout or any other), you simply increase the load gradually—maybe by just a few pounds every week or two—thus ensuring that your body is always forced to work harder. Good form is imperative here so if you have any concerns, I would recommend you hire a trainer to help. These exercises are safe with proper technique and slow, steady progression.

The bottom line is that strength and cardio fitness are both valuable areas to target when adding exercise to your life. In addition to increasing cardio activity, like walking or running, incorporating a bit of strength training into your week is well worth the effort. And it is a great place to start exercising if that is what suits you, your life, and your goals.

Variety Is the Spice of Life (and Exercise)

This is just a preliminary introduction to how you can incorporate exercise into your life. It can be as complex or as simple as you want. Whether you choose running, walking, basketball, or weight lifting, each form of exercise is beneficial to your body and to your health. Each has some specific advantages that another may not, so varying your activities from time to time will broaden your benefits and maintain your interest. Try something new once in a while, and your body will thank you for it.

Is It Safe for Me to Exercise?

A common caveat before any physical activity program is to consult your physician. Honestly, there are very few things that would make me advise a patient that it's unsafe to go for a walk or start a basic structured exercise program. The benefits of an exercise program far outweigh any risks for the vast majority of individuals.

A simple questionnaire was developed by British Columbia's Ministry of Health to help assess risk of exercise; it is now used worldwide, often by various gyms or trainers. It is called the physical activity readiness questionnaire (PAR-Q+). Keep in mind that these are screening questions meant to ensure that *no individuals are injured* with exercise at the cost of flagging some people who are really at low risk. If you answer "no" to all of the following seven questions, it is considered safe for you to start exercising.

1. Has your doctor ever said that you have a heart condition *or* high blood pressure?

2. Do you feel pain in your chest at rest, during your activities of daily living, *or* when you do physical activity?

3. Do you lose balance because of dizziness *or* have you lost consciousness in the past twelve months?

4. Have you ever been diagnosed with another chronic medical condition (other than heart disease or high blood pressure)?

5. Are you currently taking prescribed medications for a chronic medical condition?

6. Do you currently have (or have had within the past twelve months) a bone, joint, or soft tissue (muscle, ligament, or tendon) problem that could be made worse by becoming more physically active?

7. Has your doctor ever said that you should only do medically supervised physical activity?

These questions could give the impression that exercise of any kind is a risky endeavor for those with any medical condition. Realistically, it is not. The "+" was added to the PAR-Q+ to include a secondary list of questions if you answered "yes" to any of the above, in order to decrease the number of people recommended to seek clearance from their physician who were actually at low risk. If you have concerns after completing the full questionnaire, please talk to your doctor. But for the vast majority of people, increasing your exercise levels will help your overall health and likely will also have some benefit for any specific chronic health condition.

Summary

Moving—in any way you are able—is one of the simple but not easy choices to make in order to be healthier. It can be challenging to find the time and energy to increase your levels of exercise and physical activity, but it is undoubtedly one of the best things you can do for yourself. If you want to focus on one way to improve your overall health, moving more is the one to target.

All exercise and physical activity count, and the more you can do, the more benefits you will receive. Given the short-term and immediate gains you can experience—better sleep, more energy, more strength, more endurance, and decreased pain—as well as the long-term health benefits—decreased risk of death, cancer, dementia, diabetes, and heart disease—the energy spent on this aspect of health will be a great investment for yourself and your family.

So, move more, make your day harder, add exercise to your week, and add years to your life.

5

Sleep

*"Sleep is that golden chain that ties health
and our bodies together."*
Thomas Dekker

ONE OF THE most common complaints I hear in the family practice setting is fatigue. Everyone is tired and hopes that there is some simple explanation for it—low iron or low thyroid function, for example. Truthfully, only a small percentage of fatigue cases actually has a cause that can be remedied simply. For the rest, the reasons are multifactorial—some combination of issues such as stress, poor diet, lack of exercise, poor quality of sleep, and insufficient quantity of sleep.

This chapter will focus primarily on the sleep aspect of that equation, but be aware that improvements in other aspects of your life, outlined in other chapters, will also have positive effects on sleep. When it comes to health, it's all linked together.

I'm sure you have had nights where you have tossed and turned, unable to sleep soundly. Although having trouble sleeping on occasion is extremely common and normal, it is considered an issue when it becomes chronic (technically defined as three nights a week for at least three months) and affects your daily life. Insomnia is defined as the inability to sleep despite given the opportunity to do so, and it can include difficulty in falling asleep, difficulty in staying asleep, and/or waking up too early.

Insomnia is the most common type of sleep disorder in the United States, with an estimated forty million Americans experiencing it each year with 30 percent of individuals complaining of some level of sleep disruption. In Canada, approximately one-third of adults sleep less than the minimum recommendation of seven hours per night and as many as 43 percent of men and 55 percent of women complain of at least some difficulty falling or staying asleep. As my goal is to draw attention to those actions that can help improve anyone's health (rather than advise on treating specific conditions), this chapter focuses on positive sleep practices that will help those with insomnia and anyone with an occasional difficulty sleeping. There are many other potential causes of sleep disturbance (obstructive sleep apnea, restless legs syndrome, sleepwalking, teeth grinding, periodic leg movement disorder), but they are beyond the scope of this book; further medical consultation is recommended and likely required for them.

The effects of insomnia can be widespread and profound. Poor sleep can lead to excessive drowsiness, lack of energy, decreased attention, and decreased motivation—particularly when doing monotonous or boring tasks. The effects of poor sleep can then lead to an increased risk of accidents and injury—when driving, for example. In terms of overall function, however, we probably overestimate how much lack of sleep affects us; a bad night here or there really has minimal effect on our ability to do challenging work. The first thing that is noted in studies on sleep deprivation—probably to no one's surprise—is a loss of joy, followed by increased sleepiness and then grumpiness. Increased anxiety and irritability are also common in the chronically sleep-deprived.

These symptoms of fatigue, and concerns around insomnia, lead millions of people every year to spend billions of dollars on sleep aids; in the US alone, $41 billion was spent on these items in 2015.

It is estimated that one out of every two people has used tranquillizers at some point and one out of five uses them regularly. While it is understandable to want a pill to quickly fix a complex problem, it is not the answer. The actual solution requires more effort but is much more effective than any pill.

Once again, it starts with finding your reasons: Why it is worth your effort and time to improve your sleep? It is something you do every night and is clearly an important part of your health. In its favor, improving sleep has a much more immediate and direct effect on your overall feeling of well-being than making a dietary change or starting an exercise. Theoretically that should help you put in the effort to improve sleep and make it a priority, but rationality doesn't always work when it comes to making lifestyle changes. If you are struggling with fatigue and feel that an improvement in your sleep could lead to an improvement in your overall quality of life, and you feel that a better night's sleep can increase your energy for your family, your work, and your play—then I have a question for you:

Why do you deserve to make the effort to ensure that you get the best sleep you can, each and every night, to be at your best for you, your family, your job, and your life? Because ... (If you need help with your answer, check out the ignition statement section on page 40.)

How Much Sleep Do You Need?

The first thing that most people want to know when it comes to sleep is how much do humans need. We've all been told that eight hours is the magic number, but the answer is highly individual, as are most things related to sleep. On average, it seems that people tend to do better when they sleep at least seven to seven and a half hours a night. Some people can get by with less (the rare person on as few as three hours), but it is very unusual to require fewer than six hours of sleep a night. The National Sleep Foundation recommends that adults aim to get between seven and nine hours of sleep. However, it is very important to understand the variability of individual needs and figure out what is best for you—maybe you need more, maybe you need less. I have many patients who struggle with sleep solely because they worry that they aren't getting as much sleep as they *should*—even though they don't feel tired, don't need to nap, and are functioning perfectly well.

How Much Sleep Do I Get?

The best way to start improving your sleep is to gather some baseline data. Most people tend to underestimate how much sleep they get; they feel like they are tossing and turning all night but, in actuality, are asleep for a significant portion of the night. A sleep diary can help document and gain a more accurate sense of the amount of sleep you are getting and your general patterns for sleep. Thankfully, these kinds of sleep journals are not meant to be 100 percent accurate. (Determining exactly how long you are awake in the middle of the night is *not* going to help you fall asleep.) A rough estimate of the time it takes to fall asleep, the number of wake-ups, and the total time asleep will give you sufficient information to help determine strategies to improve your sleep and monitor the success of those strategies.

A sleep diary should take only a minute or two in the morning when you get up; simply estimate the times and numbers as best you can. The National Sleep Foundation has a simple diary that can be printed off and filled in.

This diary also suggests you track other factors to provide you with some excellent information about your sleep: what time you went to bed, number of wake-ups, actual sleep times, caffeine intake, medication usage, exercise, and so on. This information can be helpful to determine your sleep patterns and which factors may be influencing them. You can focus your strategies for improvement and compare your sleep to your baseline information to help quantify how much your sleep improves over time. Sleep apps are also available; many have a free version, which you could test out.

One of the most important measurements is something called your *sleep efficiency*. This is the ratio of the amount of time you are *asleep* to the amount of time you are *in bed*. It has been found that the majority of poor sleepers try to compensate for their lack of sleep by increasing their *time in bed*, which tends to decrease their efficiency and increase their frustration. I discuss sleep efficiency later in this chapter.

The Many Factors Involved in Sleep

Thankfully most of the factors that contribute to fatigue and poor sleep are consistent with the areas of focus for overall wellness. Your healthy actions do not occur in silos; a positive (or negative) behavior in one aspect of health will have similar effects on others. Below is a brief review of the main issues (other than sleep quality and quantity) and how they pertain to sleep.

Diet

When and what you eat can certainly affect your sleep. While eating a large meal may make you feel drowsy, it can also make your digestive system work too hard for you to sleep well. Try to eat a lighter meal in the evening and not too close to bedtime. Also avoid any foods that might give you heartburn or indigestion, like acidic, spicy, or greasy food. As mentioned in the "Eat" chapter, avoiding hunger is also important, so some people may require an evening snack an hour or two before bedtime. Aim for approximately 100 to 200 calories of nutrient-rich foods with some whole-grain carbohydrates and protein: some apple slices and peanut butter, a few crackers and slices of cheese, a small bowl of high-fiber cereal with skim milk, for example.

Exercise

Increased physical activity has been shown to help with sleep in a number of ways. Your increase in body temperature during exercise is followed by a compensatory drop a few hours later that seems to be conducive for sleep. It also helps to promote deeper and more restful sleep, presumably as a response to the physical stress on the body.

Caffeine

While we all likely know someone who can drink an espresso right before bed and sleep just fine, for most of us that's an easy recipe for a bad night's sleep. If insomnia is a concern at all, then it is best to limit coffee and caffeinated beverages to one or two in the morning and none after noon.

Nicotine

Smoking is a delivery mechanism for nicotine, which is a stimulant just as caffeine is. You must avoid having a cigarette in the evening or when you can't sleep at night if you are trying to sleep better. Add that to the already long list of reasons to quit smoking.

Alcohol

While alcohol can make people drowsy and help them fall asleep, the quality of sleep tends to be poor, and the quantity is also less when taking into account the multiple wake-ups overnight. A glass of wine with dinner will likely be out of your system by bedtime, but more drinks closer to sleeping will undoubtedly have a negative effect—not to mention the increased likelihood of having to get up to pee.

Stress

Many people have a hard time falling asleep due to an inability to "shut their mind off." They continually replay events of the day or go through what needs to be done tomorrow. I recommend that before bed patients make lists for the next day and most find this to be very helpful. Often, while lying in bed, your brain will continually go over your overwhelming mental list in an attempt to reduce the risk of forgetting; however, when you make a list before bed, the tasks seem much more doable, and your brain can relax as it no longer has to remember the items. Some people also find journaling before bed, or sometime in the evening, to be a useful way to get their worries off their mind and onto paper (not for anyone else to see). The simple act of organizing your worries and thoughts into a cohesive list, sentence, or paragraph can be very therapeutic.

The Case Against Sleeping Pills

Given all the above factors that have been shown to influence sleep, why are we so quick to jump to sleeping pills, either prescription or over-the-counter? In many ways, it is understandable—the desire to have a good night's sleep is so strong and the marketing of these pills suggests they're safe and effective. Why make all that effort if a pill can easily help? Unfortunately, the reality is quite different.

Do They Work?

There are two main reasons why patients want to take sleeping pills: to improve their night's sleep and to ensure good functioning the next day. When looking at the research on the effect of sleep aids on quality of sleep, the benefits seem minimal. One review found that they only improved sleep by an average of twenty-five minutes per night. Another study showed that among a group of insomniacs who took sleeping pills, the time it took to fall asleep only decreased by 4.2 minutes. So, the benefits in helping people sleep more and easier seem overstated at best.

In terms of functioning the next day, studies have repeatedly shown that taking a sleeping pill has not improved performance compared to sleeping poorly and taking a placebo pill; this has been the case with any number of tasks including math, drawing, memory, video games and decision-making. The best case is that there is no difference between taking the medication and sleeping poorly and, in most cases, it was worse—the medication stays in your system after you wake up and has an ongoing effect on your mental function (the "hangover effect").

Psychological vs. Physical Dependence

Any sleeping aid can cause some *psychological dependence*, which simply means that your body is convinced it can't sleep without it and, if you were to stop it (be it a glass of warm milk, a medication, or a herbal supplement), your insomnia would return. This *rebound insomnia* is a common occurrence and can be a factor that convinces people their medication is working and is needed, when in reality its effects are short-term and small.

Some medications seem more prone to developing *physical dependence* in some individuals; this involves the development of *tolerance* (where you need higher and higher doses to achieve the same effect) and the potential for *withdrawal* (where you experience new and different symptoms beyond insomnia when trying to stop). If you have been taking prescription sleeping pills for years (particularly a benzodiazepine—like lorazepam, clonazepam, and other -pam drugs), it is best to taper off slowly and under the guidance of your physician.

Risks, Side Effects, and Interaction

All sleeping pills have notable potential risks and side effects. Daytime drowsiness can be a risk factor in driving and increases the chance of accidents; often you are not aware that your reflexes and reaction times are slower than normal. The effects of the drug can also impair coordination and increase the risk of falls, particularly if you have to get up at night to go to the washroom or for some other reason. The combination of sleeping pills and other drugs can also have serious consequences, the most common one being alcohol and sleeping pills which together increase the risk of serious harm or even death. Avoid combining alcohol and sleeping pills.

Sleeping Pills Can Mask Other Problems

Beyond the fact that sleeping medications don't address the typical underlying issues around sleep, which we will look at shortly, they may actually hide other issues that can and do affect it. Depression can be a cause of poor sleep and it would be more effective to address that diagnosis properly via your physician rather than just taking sleeping aids. Pain is another issue that can cause people to not sleep well; taking appropriate pain medication may similarly be more effective than just an over-the-counter sleeping pill. Boredom can even be a factor in some cases in that people escape to the bedroom rather than fully interacting with others. This factor would have a different treatment plan and should be explored with your family, friends, and your physician.

When Is It Reasonable to Take a Sleeping Pill?

Despite all the negatives, there may still be a role for taking a sleeping medication in certain circumstances and under certain guidelines. There are numerous types and categories of medications available and a review of them all is beyond the scope of this book. Most of them require a prescription, so you would discuss them with your physician prior to their use. However, let's review the easily attainable over-the-counter sleep aids.

The active ingredient in most non-prescription sleeping pills and "nighttime" cold medications is an antihistamine, which is most effective for allergies. A common side effect of some medications in this class is drowsiness, and it is this side effect that is being marketed for the insomniac. There is no evidence that these medicines actually help people *sleep* better.

Melatonin is marketed as a natural product to help with sleep. It is a brain hormone that helps indicate to our body that it is dark outside. In small doses (0.3 mg), it may be useful to indicate sleep time to help with jet lag in those who do not otherwise have trouble sleeping. In higher doses (3 mg), it may help induce sleep but the evidence is not clear. It is important to be cautious with melatonin for a couple of reasons: first, because it is sold as a "health supplement," there is less regulation involved and thus you cannot be certain of its purity; second, it is a hormone with the potential for unclear effects on other body systems, including cardiovascular and reproductive systems, which is a cause for concern.

Overall, it is best to be cautious and try other avenues for sleep improvement first. If you feel you cannot avoid medications, discuss your options with your physician and keep the following in mind:

- Take the lowest dose you can.

- Use a drug with the shortest half-life or duration of action (to avoid drowsiness the next day).

- Realize that it may be appropriate to take the medication for a specific temporary crisis, such as mourning the death of a loved one, going through a divorce, or dealing with an acute medical problem.

- Take it for the shortest time possible (no longer than two to three weeks) and stop as soon as the crisis has passed.

- Avoid taking it on consecutive nights and only take it after having two bad nights in a row.

- Do not take the medication with alcohol.

- Inform your doctor if you are taking other medication.

- Never take a higher dosage than recommended by your doctor.

Some patients find the knowledge of just having a small prescription on hand helpful to their psychology of sleep. In those cases, having a small number of sleeping pills in the medicine cabinet may be of benefit.

Proper Sleep Hygiene

The topic of *sleep hygiene* refers to the habits and practices conducive to getting good sleep. People who sleep easily may not have to worry about any of these issues; but if you are having trouble with sleep, then it is worth trying to incorporate as many of them as you can. Thankfully most can be initiated quite easily, but it takes effort to be consistent. Some of the behaviors have been discussed previously and some will require some trial and error on your part to figure out what works best for you. Most aspects of sleep are highly individualized, so what works for one person may not work for another. Given that, consider the following actions and tweak them to suit you.

Set a Consistent Wake Time

When most people think about sleep, their first focus is on what time they go to sleep. In reality, it is very hard, if not impossible, to control when you fall asleep. What you can control is what time you wake up and get out of bed. You then base the rest of your planning around this wake-up time. Set an effective alarm to ensure you get up when planned, and so your body can relax knowing there is no chance of accidently sleeping in. It is also best to be consistent with this all week long; when you allow yourself to sleep in on the weekends, it makes it harder to return to your normal routine on Sunday night and you can end up starting the week frustrated with a night of poor sleep.

Set a Consistent Bedtime

While you can't set the time you actually fall asleep, it is important to set a regular bedtime. Routines are very helpful for sleep, so it is best to also go to bed at a standard time that makes sense given your set wake time. Again, try to be consistent all week long.

Create the Right Environment (for You)

Experiment with your bed and bedroom to discover in which environment you sleep best. Factors to look at include your mattress (firm/soft), your pillow (firm/soft, thick/thin), your sheets/comforter (cotton, silk, heaviness), the room temperature (cold/warm), the darkness of the room (consider blackout curtains, remove extra sources of light), how loud the room is (do you need a white noise machine?), and humidity levels. Try any changes you make for one or two weeks to see if it helps. Keeping a sleep diary during the change can also help you quantify which factors support good sleep for you.

Keep Your Bed for Sleep and Sex Only

You want to train your body to think of your bed as a place to sleep, and not as a place to watch television, work, surf the internet, have intense conversations, or play video games. Keeping your bed as a sacred space for sleep (and "recreation") will help you associate it with sleep exclusively.

Avoid Napping

It can be hard to go to sleep at a proper bedtime if you have had a nap for two hours during the day. Even if you have had a bad night, try to push through and go to bed at the same time that night. Likely you will fall asleep faster and sleep deeper to compensate.

If you do find that napping works in your lifestyle (again, sleeping is very individualistic), set an alarm, aim for less than forty-five minutes, and do not nap after four pm. Our sleep cycles tend to naturally make it easier to wake up after twenty to thirty minutes and then again after about ninety minutes. For that reason, I find if I plan for a thirty-minute nap, I usually wake up on my own before my alarm goes off; if I set it for an hour, I am woken up in the depths of my sleep cycle and feel terrible.

No Smoking

No Caffeine After Noon

Exercise Regularly

As noted earlier, exercise helps with sleep; it is best to work out in the late afternoon or early evening, not too close to bedtime. But anytime is better than never. Find something that works for you and try to do it consistently.

Avoid Heavy Meals Before Bedtime

Aim to eat a lighter meal three to four hours before bed and maybe a light snack (100–200 calories of carbohydrates and protein) one to two hours prior to bed. Again, this may require some experimentation to find what works best for you.

Turn Off Screens at least Thirty Minutes Before Bedtime

Watching television, surfing the internet, working on your phone, and checking email can all impact your ability to sleep at night. Many of these activities keep our minds busy, and it is important to give your brain some time to calm down prior to sleep. The light emitted from screens can affect melatonin levels (which are a natural trigger for sleep) and thus decrease your body's sleep signals. This is why it is better to read a book or ebook (without a backlight) rather than use a tablet or phone prior to sleep. Finally, it is also best to turn off your cell phone at night so you are not disturbed by notifications; even if you don't read those texts or emails, just knowing they are there can negatively affect your sleep.

Avoid Clock Watching

You don't need to know if you are awake at 1:30 or 4:30 a.m.—it doesn't make any difference. Try turning your clock so it faces away from you and trust that your alarm will wake you up.

Create a Bedtime Routine

It is not easy to work or be in intense activity right up until the very moment you get into bed. For this reason, it is important to create a routine to help cue your body that it is time to settle down and go to sleep. This can include a warm bath, reading something relaxing, journaling, saying your prayers, or just changing into your pyjamas and brushing your teeth. Try different routines and see what works best for you.

These simple changes and habits can have a profound effect on sleep. By implementing and targeting these issues, many people experience significant improvement in their sleep quality. Investing the time to try them is valuable for everyone but especially for those of you who are finding your bed at nighttime a negative place to be.

What Do I Do if I Can't Sleep?

If you have trouble getting to sleep, or if you wake up at night and are unable to fall back asleep easily, the consensus of sleep experts everywhere is to *not* stay in bed and to *not* just keep trying. As Peter Hauri and Shirley Linde write in their straightforward and very useful book *No More Sleepless Nights*, "The truth is the harder you try to sleep, the more likely you are to remain awake."

When you find yourself awake at night, the first thing to do, I'm sorry to say, is just get over it. It's not that big a deal. We all have had occasional nights of poor sleep and we all will have more. Often, we make our nights worse by catastrophizing and telling ourselves that our day will be ruined, work will be awful, and all our plans are shot. This type of thinking only increases our anxiety further.

I've been on-call all night and still had to work the next day: I've had my share of nights of minimal sleep. I managed to survive—I may have been grumpier than usual but I was fine. Parents have all had nights where they've been kept up with an unsettled baby or a sick kid and yet still managed to go to work the next day and function reasonably well. More obscurely, the crew of *Apollo 13* slept less than four hours a day for almost four days after the explosion damaged their ship, yet they were able to still do the complex work required to return safely to Earth. That anecdote helps me believe I can get through any of my days in comparison.

So, instead of being anxious about the next day and the perceived consequences of not being asleep, you can try relaxing in bed and realizing that rest, while not as good as sleep, is a pretty reasonable substitute and has value. If you find you need distraction in order to fall back asleep, then quietly reading in bed, listening to music or a podcast, or meditating are all good activities. For some, watching television could be an option, but this wouldn't be my first recommendation since it exposes your eyes to a screen and can be too stimulating.

If your bed has become a source of stress itself due to your history of long nights, you are best to try to strengthen the association you have with your bed and good sleep. You can try an aspect of the Bootzin technique, which was developed in the 1960s as a type of stimulus-control therapy to treat insomnia. In this technique, you focus on being in bed only for sleep: go to bed when sleepy and, if you are unable to fall asleep, get up out of bed to do something quietly (read a relaxing book, do some simple word puzzles) until you feel sleepy enough to try again. Repeat these steps as often as necessary until your body eventually associates your bed with falling asleep quickly and easily.

No matter what you decide to try with your overnight wakeups, it is best to still get up at the same time in the morning and avoid napping. You will then have a better chance of having a good sleep the next night and keep your overall sleep hygiene intact.

Sleep Restriction Therapy

If you are still struggling with sleep despite adjusting your environment, habits, and hygiene around sleep, there is another technique shown to be effective for improving sleep quality and efficiency. Sleep restriction therapy is a type of specific behavioral intervention that attempts to consolidate your broken-up night into a longer and deeper stretch of sleep by limiting your time in bed.

In a review of studies about this therapy, it was found to be at least as effective as sleeping pills and with longer-lasting effects. The downside is that it does take some dedicated effort and may initially result in more disrupted sleep and fatigue. However, with persistent effort, insomnia is significantly improved. The therapy itself is fairly straightforward and shows improved results when compared to sleep hygiene alone, and you can do this yourself without any complicated monitoring.

The steps of sleep restriction therapy are very similar to the features of good sleep hygiene but the focus is more on time in bed. Sleep restriction therapy also offers a more structured progression to foster ongoing improvement toward more restful nights.

1. Set a wake time and get up at that time regardless of how much sleep you have the night before.

2. Set your bedtime based on the average number of hours of sleep you currently get (based on your sleep diary) plus an additional thirty minutes. This may mean you are only allowed to be in bed for six hours a night initially... but it is not advised to plan for less than 5.5 hours.

3. Strictly adhere to this schedule for at least two weeks.

4. Increase your time in bed by fifteen minutes every two weeks as needed until you are sleeping well at night and feel good during the day.

5. Use bright lights (sunlight or a light box) to help trigger wakefulness in the morning, and dim lights at night to cue sleepiness.

6. Practice the other aspects of good sleep hygiene.

This technique is not for everyone. If you have significant trouble staying awake until your bedtime, do not persist with this therapy. Continue with your sleep hygiene practice and consult your physician for further support.

Summary

Having a good night's sleep and feeling energetic each and every day is a huge component of feeling well and being well. A lot of factors can be adjusted to improve sleep without having to resort to medication. These efforts can result in significantly improved sleep, which can be maintained for much longer than the effect of any pill.

However, like with any foundation of good health, it takes effort, patience, and thoughtful planning. It also takes commitment and the belief that it is worth it. You need to remind yourself of the reasons you deserve to have a good night's rest and why you deserve to make it a priority. The fact that sleep is important is no secret: you know that you feel better after a good night's sleep, you have more energy to do the things you love, and you're able to do them fully.

Be encouraged by the knowledge that you can do tangible and effective things to improve sleep right away. Work on your sleep hygiene—the practices and habits that are conducive to sleeping well. If you still have trouble, that's okay; occasional nights of poor sleep are a normal part of life. If you continue to struggle, look at the underlying causes and consider making further changes to your sleep hygiene or consider sleep restriction therapy.

Thankfully, the techniques involved in improving your sleep hygiene and overall sleep habits are straightforward to implement and can be started very easily. It may take some time to get used to the changes, but the actual interventions are not complicated and don't require fancy equipment.

If improving sleep is one of your priorities in health, then the suggestions here should give you plenty of specific ways to target your challenges, help you sleep better, and give you more energy as a result. Make the effort to sleep better and your body and mind will thank you. You deserve to live the best life you can, so remember your reasons to thrive and use that fuel to ignite your efforts to sleep better tonight.

6

Enjoy

"Happiness is a choice that requires effort at times."
Aeschylus

WHEN PEOPLE ARE asked about what they want out of life, they often mention things like cars, a big house, travel, money, and more leisure time at first, but eventually they come to the heart of it: they just want to be happy. In fact, all of those other wishes are pursued in an ongoing quest for happiness.

Ultimately, that seems to be what we all desire and struggle with each and every day: "How can I be happier in this moment and in this life?"

It is what we wish for our children: "I just want them to be happy."

It is what we want for our friends and family: "Here's wishing you health and happiness..."

Health and happiness. That's all we really want, isn't it? But they aren't two separate things; they are interrelated. It is harder to be happy if you are struggling with your health, and it's harder to be healthy if you aren't enjoying your life.

Health and happiness are the two great equalizers in society—it doesn't matter if you are rich and famous if you are also unwell and miserable.

Evidence supports the idea that material wealth isn't everything. Studies have shown that the wealthy are not much happier than the average person, with one study showing that there was no difference in day-to-day happiness beyond an annual income of approximately $75,000. Daniel Kahneman, a Nobel Prize winner in economics who went on to research happiness, made the following comment regarding wealth and positive emotions:

> The belief that high income is associated with good mood is widespread but mostly illusory. People with above-average income are relatively satisfied with their lives but are barely happier than others in moment-to-moment experience, tend to be more tense, and do not spend more time in particularly enjoyable activities. Moreover, the effect of income on life satisfaction seems to be transient. We argue that people exaggerate the contribution of income to happiness because they focus, in part, on conventional achievements when evaluating their life or the lives of others.

In general, once our basic financial needs are met (food, housing, security), wealth does not seem to affect our baseline rates of happiness. And what are these "conventional achievements" Kahneman is referring to? These are the typical trappings of success—cars, vacations, clothes, toys, houses— that we expect to make us happy but which really don't.

Is Happiness the Same as Pleasure?

It is also easy to be confused between pleasure and happiness. *Pleasure* is defined as a feeling of satisfaction and enjoyment. You would think that feeling this way more often would make you happier, and it may... but it may not. While it can be valuable and motivating, pleasure is transient and not enough to drive *happiness* itself. The constant pursuit of pleasure and the expectation that you should strive to be in a constant state of joy is unrealistic and will undoubtedly lead to disappointment. Though it is not possible to be happy if there is no joy or pleasure in your life, pleasure alone *is not enough*.

Another view that can lead you astray is the idea that happiness is some destination in the future. "I will be happy when... I graduate, get that job, get that promotion, buy that house, go on that trip, make that team, win that championship, get married, have kids, the kids leave, when I retire." Happiness isn't something to strive for in the distance but rather something to work for now. Every day you can work toward being happier than you were yesterday.

One simple definition of happiness is experiencing frequent positive emotions (joy, interest, pride) and infrequent *but not absent* negative emotions (sadness, anger, anxiety). This characterization effectively expresses that it is a *general state* of happiness rather than a specific moment. I appreciate how Sonja Lyubomirsky—positive psychology researcher, professor of psychology at the University of California, and author of *The How of Happiness*—defines happiness as "the experience of joy, contentment, or positive well-being, combined with the sense that one's life is good, meaningful, and worthwhile."

This aspect of *meaning* is an important one that differentiates true happiness from simple pleasure. If our personal pursuits are in keeping with our intrinsic values and goals, then they provide joy in a different way than hedonistic pursuits. We are able to delay gratification and tolerate periods of hardship, challenge, or boredom as we follow our ultimate objectives. In an extreme example, Viktor Frankl, author of the classic book *Man's Search for Meaning,* was a psychiatrist who was imprisoned in three different concentration camps during World War II and endured the loss of his entire family, torture, humiliation, and unimaginable hardships. He found a way to survive emotionally by focusing on his personal purpose. Even through those horrendous atrocities, he found some meaning for his life.

It would be a stretch to say that Frankl was "happy" during that period, but his outlook shows the power of finding meaning. What we strive for is a combination of pleasure coupled with an intrinsic value and purpose for our life. Working together, they can be a powerful synergistic union that provides fuel for our days. As Tal Ben-Shahar says in his book *Happier,* "When we derive a sense of purpose from what we do, our experience of pleasure is intensified; and taking pleasure in an activity can make our experience of it all the more meaningful."

Seeing that you now have a very general sense of what happiness is, are there tangible ways to work toward it? Thankfully the evidence shows that there is. Studies also demonstrate that improving happiness seems to improve health in a variety of ways beyond just the emotional benefits. Despite this evidence, most people do not think about their level of happiness as they would their weight or fitness level. People will try lots of diets and exercise programs in a quest for wellness but seem to be much less likely to invest in the practices that have been shown to be helpful in increasing happiness. Yet happiness is a key factor in your health, and I'm sure many would choose being happy over being healthy—I like to think you can do both.

Benefits of Improved Happiness

As research into happiness increases, more and more evidence shows the benefits of being happier. The first benefit is... being happier. I mean, who doesn't want to have a generally better outlook on life, feel more grateful for the life they have, and experience more positive emotions than negative ones?

But beyond that there are some incredible tangible benefits shown to be related to levels of happiness. Let's review a few of them.

Increased Longevity

In an interesting study, researchers from the University of Kentucky found a pile of handwritten autobiographies that nuns wrote upon entering the convent in the 1930s and 1940s. The researchers found it wasn't difficult to sort these journals into four categories based on a continuum of negative to positive emotion. The incredible thing about studying this group of nuns is that their lives were very consistent—in terms of diet, activity, sleep, relationships, environment, activities, stressors, and smoking status—which are very hard to control in any typical research project. They then found these women decades later and were able to compare the groups at different times. They discovered some astonishing associations between their mood and longevity:

- Nuns in the most positive category lived on average *ten years longer* than those in the most negative category.

- By age eighty, the happiest group had lost 25 percent of its members compared to the least happy group, which had lost 60 percent.

* Only 34 percent of the lowest mood category reached the age of eight-five as opposed to 90 percent of the highest mood category.

It seems that finding ways to be happier could add years to your life and enjoyment to your years. That type of intervention definitely seems to be worth the effort.

Strengthened Immune System

Patients are always wondering about ways to boost their immune system with diet changes, vitamins, and supplements. I usually recommend sleeping well, washing hands often, eating more fruits and vegetables, and keeping your vaccinations up-to-date. It seems that improving happiness levels should be added to that list. A study in 2003 took 350 adults and sadistically exposed them to the common cold virus. In the two weeks prior to that, they were called several times and asked how much they had experienced several positive emotions. The results of the study showed that those who had scored higher in that regard were less likely to contract the cold despite exposure to the virus.

Apparently getting a cold can make you feel miserable, but feeling miserable may make you more prone to catching a cold.

Improved Heart Health

Happiness levels also seem to relate to the health of your heart. Various studies have shown correlation between feeling happier and having better readings in regards to blood pressure, resting heart rate, and heart rate variability. In the 1995 Nova Scotia Health Survey, more than 1,700 adults were assessed on a five-point scale for positive emotions and followed for ten years. The results found that those with a higher rating in regards to happiness had a 22 percent lower chance of experiencing a heart attack. It seems that a happy heart may well be a healthier heart.

Decreased Pain

Chronic pain is a common issue that many have to learn how to manage and endure. Several studies show that having a positive mood and a higher level of happiness can decrease levels of pain. A study of more than 1,000 people dealing with arthritis found that those with higher happiness scores had less pain and walked more steps each day. Another study looking at 1,000 people recovering from stroke found that those with a more positive outlook had significantly lower pain ratings three months after the event. Other studies also show this trend and, while it's not clear how happiness levels lessen pain, it is another worthwhile reason to try to improve the level of joy in our lives.

Increased Resilience

Resilience is defined as the ability to recover quickly from difficulties or challenges. Resilience helps you pull through periods of stress and unexpected problems, and increased levels of happiness seem to be associated with increased levels of this valuable trait. It is actually hard to know if happiness increases resilience or if it's the other way around, but they are interrelated. Feeling more positive and having more experiences where you have recovered from challenges improves your ability to do that in the future and thus improves your likelihood of bouncing back and your overall outlook on life. They seem to build on each other in a very beneficial way.

Given these significant benefits to being happier, the next question is whether or not it is possible to change our baseline level of happiness. Thankfully, the answer seems to be yes!

Set Point Theory of Happiness

People tend to have a certain level of happiness that seems to be determined by genetics and by childhood experiences. This set point, much like the set temperature on a thermostat, offsets external changes, thus bringing people back to their general outlook despite changes in external factors, like winning the lottery or dealing with a health crisis. We also have seen that people who are happier, or who have higher set points, seem to have numerous health benefits. Researchers set out to see if it is possible to *increase* this happiness set point.

Lyubomirsky, author of *The How of Happiness*, determined through her research that 50 percent of our happiness level is determined by our genes, 10 percent by the circumstances of our life, and *40 percent by our voluntary actions and choices*. Given that, it is exciting to think about how much potential we have to adjust our outlook through our personal decisions.

A study of 150,000 Germans over twenty-five years, looking at their life satisfaction and other aspects of happiness, seemed to show this to be the case. Over the course of the study, people were able to change their percentile ranking in terms of happiness quite significantly; a quarter of people improved their position by 33 percent or more, and 12 percent by over 50 percent. These findings certainly suggest that your set point of happiness is not fixed in stone and can be altered over time.

Further research by Lyubomirsky showed an example of *how* to achieve that change in positive outlook. She asked students to do five acts of kindness each week for six weeks and, over the course of the study, the students who performed more acts of kindness showed a significant increase in their levels of happiness compared to those in the control group. This finding again supports the idea that our personal choices can improve the level of satisfaction in our lives.

Positive Psychology

Positive psychology is a relatively new field within psychology that focuses on those strengths and factors that enable individuals and communities to thrive and flourish. This outlook was originated by Dr. Martin Seligman in 1998, and it uses science to look at the issues that help people become happier rather than looking at how to make people feel less sad.

Depression is unfortunately one of the most common conditions we treat in medicine. If you are feeling depressed to the point that you are feeling significant dysfunction in regards to work, relationships, and life in general, you should seek medical help. While the field of happiness research can still be useful for those with clinical depression, it is not meant to replace medical support. There is a clear difference between the goal of getting people out of the depths of depression and the goal of helping people become happier.

The patient health questionnaire (PHQ-9) is a multipurpose tool that many physicians use to screen and monitor depression. It uses some diagnostic criteria and common depression symptoms, along with their frequency and severity, to create a score that can be tracked over time.

THE PATIENT HEALTH QUESTIONNAIRE (PHQ-9)

Over the past two weeks, how often have you been bothered by any of the following problems?	Not at all	Several days	More than half the days	Nearly every day
Little interest or pleasure in doing things?	0	1	2	3
Feeling down, depressed, or hopeless?	0	1	2	3

Over the past two weeks, how often have you been bothered by any of the following problems?	Not at all	Several days	More than half the days	Nearly every day
Trouble falling asleep, staying asleep, or sleeping too much?	0	1	2	3
Feeling tired or having little energy?	0	1	2	3
Poor appetite or overeating?	0	1	2	3
Feeling bad about yourself—or that you're a failure or have let yourself or your family down?	0	1	2	3
Trouble concentrating on things, such as reading the newspaper or watching television?	0	1	2	3
Moving or speaking so slowly that other people could have noticed? Or the opposite—being so fidgety or restless that you have been moving around a lot more than usual?	0	1	2	3
Thoughts that you would be better off dead or of hurting yourself in some way?	0	1	2	3
Total				

My point in showing this questionnaire is only to note that if you were to score zero, it would only indicate that you were not depressed, but it would do *absolutely nothing* to indicate your level of happiness. It is not a health or happiness question-naire; it is a tool to monitor clinical depression. This emphasis on the negative has been the trend of much of psychology and psychiatry over the past decades, and this shift toward positive aspects of psychology—including how we can develop our own happiness—is a welcome change.

This new outlook provides a much more active approach to mental well-being with research into tools and activities every-one can do to improve overall happiness and life satisfaction.

It is exciting to think of all the tangible things you can do to improve the joy and happiness in your life, especially when considering that only 10 percent of your life satisfaction is due to circumstances and a full 40 percent is in your control. But before we get into the proven actions you can take to increase the joy and positive satisfaction in your life, I have another question for you.

Why do you deserve to be happier? Why should you make the efforts to enjoy life more and truly feel happier—tomorrow, next week, next month, and next year—than you do today? Because... (Refer to the ignition statement section on page 40)

How to Increase Your Happiness

Research in positive psychology has discovered many actions and behaviors that are associated with, and seem to improve, the satisfaction people feel about their lives. These choices do not require a lot of fancy equipment but just a focus on making true happiness—*increased feelings of contentment and joy coupled with the sense that life is worthwhile and has meaning*—a priority. Increasing your happiness is another avenue you can take to improve your health and overall quality of life. Try to add as many of these features into your life as you can.

Find Meaning and Purpose in Your Life

There are many ways people find value and direction in their lives, but those who have a clear purpose seem to be able to handle stress better and navigate the trials and tribulations of life. They feel more in control of their lives and are more motivated in their daily actions. This meaning can look different for different people and can take various forms: being the best parent you can be; having a religious faith; being passionate about your career; or taking part in a social cause you feel strongly about.

It may take some time to find your particular source for meaning, but it is worth reflecting on what activities, people, and projects make you feel passionate and engaged. Then make sure you prioritize your time to incorporate them into your life.

You can also take the time to create your own personal mission statement. This is not the same as your ignition statement—which we discussed in "Change"—that captured *why* you do what you do; a mission statement is meant to help direct you in terms of *what* exactly you do. Stephen Covey, author of *The 7 Habits of Highly Effective People*, encourages people to create their own mission statement as a backbone for their lives. He suggests, "Writing or reviewing a mission statement changes you because it forces you to think through your priorities deeply, carefully, and to align your behavior with your beliefs."

FranklinCovey's mission statement builder is a great free online tool to prompt you to think about those things that are truly the most important to you. It takes only fifteen to forty-five minutes to complete, depending on how long you reflect on each question.

Focus on Gratitude

We all have much to be grateful for but it seems we humans are hardwired to focus on the negative. I'm not alone in how easily I can remember the times I screwed up or made a fool of myself but find it much harder to remember the times when I did a good job or someone did something nice for me. This isn't by accident: as humanity evolved, being aware of any possible dangers to our survival was an important protective feature so we learned to emphasize the negative. In order to counteract this tendency, cultivating a sense of gratitude has been found to be very beneficial in helping us even the score and focus on the positive.

A simple way to incorporate gratitude is to take a few minutes at bedtime to think about three positive things that happened during the day. It could be as simple as receiving a compliment, someone saying "thank you," participating in a hobby you love, talking to a friend, enjoying the sunshine, someone helping you with a problem, or helping someone else with a challenge. Reflecting on gratitude is also a nice technique to incorporate with children to start them focusing on the positive.

A more structured way to do this is to keep a gratitude journal by your bedside. Take a few minutes at the end of the day to write down some things you are thankful for and some positive events that occurred. By consciously choosing to focus on the positive, you can start seeing the many good things in the world that you may have been previously missing.

Be Kind to Others

Some of the best evidence regarding happiness revolves around the value of doing random acts of kindness. In his book *Flourish*, Dr. Seligman wrote, "We scientists have found that doing a kindness produces the single most reliable momentary increase in well-being of any exercise we have tested."

These studies have fine-tuned that recommendation and generated some guidelines that are worth considering:

- Any kindness (large or small) is effective, so pick something that speaks to you and makes sense for you, your family, and your life.

- Try to do something that takes you out of your routine— something you wouldn't do normally.

- Try a variety of acts of kindness, so you don't lose the positive feeling from the endeavor.

- Happy givers are likely to give more and continue to give, and the recipients tend to benefit more. It is worth finding a cause or activity that fits your personal goals and that you find some immediate joy in as well.

- One other point is that any act of kindness is meant to help others and not just yourself; while the act may temporarily be at the expense of your own immediate happiness, it has still been shown to increase your overall levels of happiness. However, ensure you maintain a balance so that you don't become a martyr—unhappy and resentful.

Savor the Joys of Life

In this hectic and fast-paced world, it can be hard to slow down and appreciate all the truly wonderful things that make life worth living. Staying in the moment and savoring— enjoying an experience slowly in order to enjoy it as much as possible—is an amazing way to experience some of life's best moments.

Mindfulness and mindfulness meditation is a skill that is very useful in this area. Being mindful is all about being present in the moment and learning to stay present despite the chaos around you. Being present allows you to enjoy the ordinary pleasures of the taste of a great meal, the smell outside after the rain, or the feel of a hot shower.

Savoring also involves remembering and reminiscing about experiences. I'm sure we can all recall the joy felt in joking with friends after a day spent on a hike, at a festival or other outing, or the pleasure of being with old friends and thinking about the fun had as kids together. Taking the time to reflect positively on good times, recent or otherwise, seems to boost your emotions in the present. So, replay, reminisce, and remember—it's worthwhile and enjoyable.

Find Your Flow

Mihaly Csikszentmihalyi, psychologist and author of *Flow: The Psychology of Optimal Experience*, describes the concept of flow—the intense absorption and involvement with the present moment—as "being completely involved in an activity for its own sake." It's the kind of activity where you are so completely absorbed in it, you lose track of time and could be unaware of hunger, thirst, or the need to use the washroom.

These kinds of activities have a clear objective and are a perfect match between the level of skill you have and the challenge of the task. If the activity is too easy, then you are bored; if your expertise is insufficient, then you may become anxious. But if you are in balance with the activity, then you are in flow. Common examples that are conducive to flow include playing an instrument, playing a sport, reading a book, writing a paper, cooking, and talking with friends. However, any activity can be made into a flow-type activity by either decreasing the difficulty or increasing your skill level.

To improve your overall levels of happiness, try to find more ways to incorporate a flow state into your life. Here are some suggestions:

- Be sure to continually learn new things—be it an instrument, a language, a topic, a sport, a game, or a recipe.

- Rediscover activities that used to make time fly by for you and make it a priority to find time for them in your week.

- Reevaluate your current state of flow. Many are surprised to realize that they are actually happier, more fulfilled, and more in flow at work when they are challenged and engaged, as opposed to in their leisure activities when they are not using their skills at all (watching Netflix, surfing the internet, or reading trashy novels).

- Honor your need to decompress, but limit your time in vegetative activities; forty-five to sixty minutes daily is likely enough.

One word of caution regarding flow: some activities that can create flow can be obviously addictive and have negative consequences (video games and gambling, for example). Even activities that seem positive (working on a project, volunteering for a charity, learning a new instrument) can lead to neglecting personal responsibilities and the needs of your loved ones. Be aware of the power of flow.

Exercise

Not to belabor the point, but yet another benefit of exercise of any kind is an improvement in mood and happiness. There is a reason why exercise is considered to be such a fantastic health intervention. Consult the "Move" chapter for tips on how to incorporate exercise into your life.

Connect with People

Having close friendships, relationships, and a strong social network is a common feature of happy people. These connections help fulfill our desire to be part of a social unit. Your social network also provides support in times of stress and need, as well as an outlet to share joy, celebrate success, and reminisce about good times.

One of the main strategies in this area is to make time for relationships. Increase the quality time you spend each week with your partner (watching television together typically doesn't count) to allow for communication and sharing. Make time for your friends as well; while many people feel some guilt around leaving their family or other obligations to spend time with friends, ensuring you have time to fill this important bucket of happiness will improve the energy and mood you have for your family and work as well.

Be Content and Don't Compare

The last way to foster happiness that I'd like to convey to you is to be more compassionate to yourself. We are often much harder on ourselves than we would ever be to others. Give yourself a break. None of us is perfect and we all have flaws that we need to be okay with.

Within this idea, there are a few concepts that are worth defining and distinguishing. Self-esteem is the feeling of how good and valuable you are, which is typically based on your performance in certain areas. Self-acceptance is more general and involves understanding your strengths and weaknesses, accepting your past, and feeling content with yourself while still being aware of your limitations. Self-compassion focuses on the behaviors and actions that foster self-acceptance: being kind and understanding to yourself; recognizing that pain and failure are unavoidable parts of the human experience; and being able to face your painful thoughts and feelings without judgment.

So be nice to yourself. Don't just treat others as you wish to be treated; treat yourself as you would treat others too. This outlook will lead to better self-esteem and higher self-acceptance. It also will help you lessen the tendency to compare yourself to others, which is particularly detrimental to your mental health. This is a common problem today when social media provides a constant source of judgment.

Action for Happiness, a movement committed to building a happier and more caring society, notes that "so often we compare our insides to other people's outsides." I think that is a great observation which highlights the challenges of living in our world of social media. We are constantly looking at our friends' posts and pictures of their "perfect" exterior life and comparing it to our imperfect lives—it's a losing battle we need to avoid. While avoiding all social media is probably not a feasible solution, limiting your exposure to it and "unfriending" those people whose posts make you feel sad or inferior is probably a good idea.

As you can see, there are many tangible actions you can take to improve your happiness. By making happiness a priority and incorporating some of these ideas into your life, you can add "being happier" to your overall health plan.

Stress Management Strategies

While many of the practices in this chapter aim to increase enjoyment, they can also be used as ways to reduce stress. In addition, there are other targeted ways to reduce stress in your busy life.

Increase Your Sense of Control

One of the biggest factors in how stressed you feel is the level of control you feel you have over your situation, be it at work or at home. Find ways to increase this control by asking for more autonomy at work, by learning new skills to address weaknesses, or getting clarity to decrease any uncertainty.

Simplify Your Life

Our lives can easily get cluttered with activities, obligations, and stuff. Look to minimize your life in any way you can to focus on what matters. This could involve limiting your possessions to what you truly love, your time commitments, your screen time, and your relationships. Focus on spending your time and energy on the people and things that add value to your life.

Improve Your Time Management

Multitasking is a myth in that you can't truly do more than one thing at a time; you just switch back and forth quickly. Even computers use high processing speeds to do this and are equally unable to do multiple activities at exactly the same time! Develop a system to help organize your time better. *Time Management from the Inside Out* by Julie Morgenstern and *Getting Things Done* by David Allen are two great resources.

Just Say No

Once you clarify your priorities and your personal mission statement, it becomes easier to decline activities that don't align with your goals. Direct your energy and excitement toward what you really care about.

Decreasing your stress levels can be a challenge, but these strategies—along with focusing on the other ways to increase your enjoyment in your life—can make a huge difference to your overall outlook. And the serenity prayer is always a good backbone for any stress management strategy, regardless of spiritual or religious outlook:

"God grant me the serenity to accept the things I cannot change, courage to change the things I can, and the wisdom to know the difference."

Summary

Enjoyment is a key ingredient to a healthy life. We've reviewed what true happiness looks like and the many benefits being happier convey to our well-being.

We've also seen how research into positive psychology and the science of how we feel happier has shown that 40 percent of our outlook on life comes from our own personal choices and behaviors. This figure provides a huge potential for actively improving our levels of happiness.

Rather than passively accepting your situation and state of mind, you now have the knowledge to consciously choose to make concrete changes and add specific activities to increase your enjoyment of life. Emphasize actions that help you:

- find meaning and purpose,
- focus on gratitude,
- be kind to others,
- savor the joys of life,
- find your flow,
- exercise,
- connect with people, and
- be content and don't compare.

It is definitely possible for you to increase the joy you experience, so make it a priority to live happier and healthier.

7

Quit

"It's not just that it's bad for you. Do you want to spend
the rest of your life fighting a stupid addiction to a stupid thing
that doesn't even really give you a good buzz?"
Katherine Heigl

"QUIT" REFERS TO one thing you should do immediately to improve your health: quit smoking. If you are currently smoking, then removing this addiction from your life is one of the best things you can do to keep your risk of heart disease, stroke, emphysema, dementia, cancer, and other illnesses low—as well as improve your health overall. And if you don't currently smoke, don't start! But you will still benefit from reading this chapter to ensure you don't ever get the urge and to better understand and help any loved ones who do smoke.

I am not a smoker and never have been. Even though I regularly see patients about their nicotine habit, understand the recommendations to help people quit, and prescribe medications as a means of helping them, I know that I am unable to grasp the magnitude of the hold nicotine has on people. I don't feel that I have to quit smoking myself in order to help people, just as I don't need to have diabetes to help manage that condition. However, when it comes to nicotine and its complex place in society, I think it is worth considering the path that ex-smokers have taken to quit to see what we can learn from their experiences.

There are a number of ways that former smokers have overcome their nicotine addiction. The most common method is quitting on their own; approximately *90 percent* of smokers who quit successfully did so with no external help. Although this is promising, when looked at reversely, only about 5 percent of smokers who try to quit cold turkey—through willpower alone—sustain their nonsmoking status for at least six to twelve months. Adding support via nicotine replacement therapy or medications seems to at least double that chance of success.

There is a school of thought that says there is a significant difference between attempting to quit using the strength of your willpower and stopping smoking when you finally accept the absurdity of smoking given its negative effects on health. While they both involve stopping smoking with no outside aids, they come from two very different mindsets with the latter requiring very little willpower as there is no feeling of missing something. Although this sounds too easy, I am sure we all have known a long-term smoker who one day decided to quit and succeeded with no apparent struggle and no supportive therapy. I've seen it numerous times among my patients; even my father decided to stop smoking on his own in his sixties after a lifetime of smoking. Other patients get to this point after a particular health scare or event, when they finally realize that the pros (which are debatable) of smoking were miniscule compared to the cons.

If you are a smoker, quitting is probably the most difficult adjustment that you will need to make. How can some people quit so easily? In reality, it likely wasn't quick for them at all but took lots of processing of information, over many years, to reach that point. What looked like a sudden realization from the outside actually took a fair amount of time.

In psychology and medicine, we typically map the process of any substantial lifestyle modification as following these stages of change:

1. *Precontemplation*—one is not even considering making the change.

2. *Contemplation*—one is starting to think about making the change but is not ready to do so yet.

3. *Preparation*—one makes plans and gets ready to make the change.

4. *Action*—one is actually making the change.

5. *Maintenance*—one is sustaining the change and preventing return to the previous behavior.

As a doctor, I try to help advance patients through these stages by providing information to increase the belief in the *importance* of quitting smoking and by providing the skills and tools to increase *confidence* in success in an attempt to quit. While it is unusual to see a person move from stage one to four in a single office visit, conversation, or discussion, it can occur quickly at times. Some people may have an epiphany because of a health scare or on a milestone birthday, decide to stop smoking, and suddenly move from contemplation to action.

Rather than using that typical model, I believe it all comes down to what we discussed in "Change": the three areas to address when making any lifestyle modification—that image of a rider on an elephant moving down a path.

Motivating the elephant is the first step: you have to *feel* the need to change and find your specific and personal reasons to quit smoking. The elephant is not rational, so simple facts are typically not enough to guide it. And without a feeling behind the intention, the chance of success is low. It's key to understand the *importance* of quitting but, more crucially, why it is important for *you*.

The rider needs to provide clear direction, which means a plan as to *how* you will eliminate smoking from your life. This plan may be as simple as "just stop smoking" but also could include nicotine replacement therapy, medication, seminars, or other techniques. A plan increases your confidence in your ability to quit smoking.

Finally, shape the path to prepare for a life without cigarettes. This could include avoiding triggers, anticipating challenges when you may crave smoking, creating new relationships (with exercise, gum, stress balls) to replace the old relationship with cigarettes, and/or the involvement of supportive counseling. A support group or coach can help to remind you of the reasons you quit and how to avoid a relapse into smoking.

Let's look at each of these factors in more detail to provide specifics for each to help guide your thought process toward a life without smoking.

Motivate the Elephant

Finding reasons to quit smoking should be easy. Everyone knows that smoking is bad for your health and that if you want to be healthy, there really is no place for cigarettes in your life. Clearly this fact is not as effective of a motivator as you'd hope; if it were, we wouldn't need those ugly pictures on cigarette packs.

But I wouldn't feel I was doing my job if I didn't at least briefly discuss the many harmful effects smoking has on your overall health. Knowing the risks is the first (and likely most ineffective) way of trying to motivate the elephant to change.

Negative Health Effects of Smoking

Smoking essentially harms every single organ system in the body. The list of conditions for which smokers have a higher risk is too long to list here, but here are some of the highlights:

- increased risk of heart attacks and strokes
- increased risk of emphysema
- increased risk of cancer of almost all types (one-third of all cancer deaths are linked to tobacco use)
- increased risk of vascular disease
- increased risk of erectile dysfunction
- increased aging and wrinkling of skin
- weakened immune system
- increased risk of dementia

The negative health issues associated with smoking are well known and numerous, but, as we've seen, not a strong motivator for quitting. So, the next avenue to consider is all of the potential benefits of quitting.

Benefits of Quitting Smoking

Whenever we talk about stopping smoking, we tend to use the term "quitting." Fair enough, but the term implies that you are giving up something, sacrificing something, or depriving yourself of something. It may be more useful to think of the situation as finding a way to *escape from* smoking or perhaps *free yourself* from smoking. You aren't just moving away from a life of smoking but rather *toward* a life as a nonsmoker. And when you make that transition, there are numerous immediate, short-term, and long-term advantages you can appreciate.

1. Improved Finances

In Canada, the cost of a pack-a-day habit is approximately $3,500 a year. While most smokers will say that they can afford it, or it's their choice to spend their money in that way, few have considered the reality that, in order to finance that cost, they will have to *earn* approximately twice that in additional pre-tax income. That can add up to $140,000 of income spent on cigarettes over the course of a twenty-year habit. What else could you do with all of that money?

2. Improved Health Function

When you smoke, you often don't realize the strong effect your habit has on you. Your breathing, energy, circulation, and heart function are all poorer as a result, but it has become your new normal—you don't realize the cigarette is one major factor causing you to not feel your best. For some reason, we tend to think of the negative health effects of smoking as black or white issues: you get cancer or you don't; you have a heart attack or you don't; you develop emphysema or you don't. We don't think about all the immediate effects that cigarettes are having on your body right now. Once you stop smoking, your body can finally start healing itself and attempt to reverse the damage being done.

- Within *twenty minutes* of your last puff, your body begins working to offset the effects of the toxins in the cigarette, and your heart rate and blood pressure start to improve.

- Within *twelve hours*, the level of carbon monoxide, which is poisonous and deadly and increased in your bloodstream when you smoke, drops down to normal.

- In only *three days*, there is no more nicotine in your body.

- In *two weeks to three months*, your circulation and lung function improve (you may cough more as your body attempts to clear out your lungs).

- In *one to nine months*, that cough settles down and your breathing also improves.

Quitting smoking gives your body a chance to heal and you a chance to realize how good you can feel without those toxins in the way. These benefits occur fairly quickly and are things you will notice; you'll feel better and have more energy for your work and family—sooner rather than later.

3. Long-term Health Benefits

Beyond those immediate improvements in health function, once you become a nonsmoker, the risk you have for that laundry list of diseases associated with smoking starts to drop right away. But let's jump right to the most basic of things we wish to delay: death. A smoker who quits before the age of forty will reduce their risk of dying from a smoking-related illness by about 90 percent. If you quit between the ages of forty-five and fifty-four, that risk is dropped by about two-thirds.

In terms of specific illnesses, here is a breakdown of how long after quitting your risks drop:

- At *one year*, your risk of heart disease is cut in half.

- At *two to five years*, your risk of mouth, throat, esophagus, and bladder cancers is cut in half; your risk of stroke is the same as a nonsmoker.

- At *ten years*, you are half as likely to die from lung cancer as a current smoker; your risk of pancreatic or kidney cancer decreases significantly.

* At *fifteen years*, you have the same risk of heart disease as a nonsmoker.

These risks start dropping the moment you escape from your nicotine habit, so the sooner you can do that, the sooner you can reduce the threats to your health caused by smoking.

For the nonsmoker, these reasons can seem like more than enough of a push to quit smoking, which can perpetuate the judgment that anyone who smokes is foolish or unintelligent to do so. That's not fair. I doubt any smoker smoked their first cigarette with the intention of becoming a life-long smoker knowing all of the long-term negative effects of smoking.

This is a great example where the Think-Analyze-Change model does not work: smokers can be presented with overwhelming evidence and data to highlight the negative consequences of smoking, but they don't seem motivated to quit. Why is that? Likely because these consequences don't address the reality of why people smoke.

Smoking Is a Nicotine Addiction

In truth, smoking is an addiction to nicotine; there are no two ways around it. Each cigarette is a nicotine-delivery device. If you smoke twenty cigarettes a day and take about fifteen puffs on each, that is 300 hits a day of this drug. Even the way people smoke has changed to maximize the size of the hit. Most people used to smoke with the cigarette dangling between their index and middle fingers and puffing casually; now many smokers hold it like a dart and suck strongly when smoking to increase the amount of the drug they get per dose.

The strangest thing about this addiction is that there really is no "high" to the drug. While there is a clear effect with strong drugs like heroin, the first sensation when smoking a cigarette is typically negative. I don't recall any patient, friend, or acquaintance who recalls that first cigarette being anything but gross. But due to the addictive potential of nicotine, that one cigarette can quickly lead to another and soon to a lifetime struggle with nicotine addiction.

And that is what smoking is—an addiction. It is not truly a habit like chewing your fingernails or cracking your knuckles. A *habit* is defined as an acquired behavior that is regularly followed until it becomes involuntary. While that could sound a bit like smoking, what fits better are the four Cs of *addiction*:

1. *Craving*
2. Loss of *control* in amount and frequency of use
3. *Compulsion* to use
4. Use despite *consequences*

Now we have an opportunity to use the See-Feel-Change model—where a smoker is faced with information or a situation that causes them to truly feel a personal reason to change and quit. The best route I can think of is to demonstrate that the *only* benefit a smoker gets from smoking is to relieve the feelings of stress, anxiety, and tension associated with the *withdrawal from their last cigarette*. That is it. The rest is all myth and advertising—it isn't cool, it doesn't relax you, it doesn't help you concentrate, it doesn't relieve boredom, and it doesn't relieve stress. All it does is relieve the withdrawal from nicotine.

Once you truly feel and believe that the only reason you smoke is to avoid withdrawal, then the actual quitting (or escape from addiction) process can be fairly easy and painless. Consider the numerous cases of people who quit with seemingly no issue at all after a health scare, the birth of a child or grandchild, or after getting to the point where enough is enough.

As I stated earlier, I'm not a smoker but one experience where I felt a similar epiphany was with my relationship to pharmaceutical representatives. I had never felt comfortable talking with them, attending their lunches, or going to educational seminars hosted by them. But I felt it was part of my job as a physician to be informed on new drugs, get samples for my patients who may have trouble affording them, and to stay connected with the medical community at large.

Then one night I tried watching the movie *Love & Other Drugs*. In the introductory scenes, the main character (played by Jake Gyllenhaal) is hired by a pharmaceutical company and is trained to become a successful drug rep. For the first time, I *saw and felt* that I was just being manipulated by these companies; I felt so agitated that I had to turn off the movie. From then on, I have been refusing to talk to industry and I feel extremely confident in that decision. I am grateful for the work that pharmaceutical companies do to develop new drugs, but I will wait for them to become the standard of care through clinical practice and not worry about being the first to use them based on their sales techniques.

That sudden and embarrassing awareness of being fooled and manipulated by a large, powerful industry is how I would expect a smoker to feel when they finally realize that the reasons they think they smoke are wrong. So let's look at some of these reasons and how they relate to the reality of the drug addiction.

The Myths of Why You Smoke

As I mentioned above, the primary physiological reason people smoke is to offset the feeling of withdrawal from nicotine. A puff of a cigarette delivers nicotine to your brain in about ten seconds. After your cigarette, there is enough nicotine in your system to keep the cravings at bay for about forty-five minutes. Doing the math explains why most smokers need about twenty to twenty-five cigarettes a day.

As the level of nicotine drops in your system, you start to feel slightly restless as if something is missing. As that feeling grows, it may lead to irritability and anxiousness. Every cigarette is used to get rid of this withdrawal and get back to feeling normal—which is how a nonsmoker feels all the time!

There is no high and there is no buzz; there is only the absence of a negative feeling. This absence can feel different to smokers at different times, but the "positive" feelings smokers associate with their cigarettes are solely due to the removal of the withdrawal symptoms. Let's look at a few examples of how this is misinterpreted.

- *Smoking helps relieve boredom.* When you are bored, you are more likely aware of the symptoms of withdrawal and therefore more likely to have a cigarette.

- *Smoking helps concentration.* When you need to concentrate, withdrawal symptoms are an additional distraction so a cigarette helps remove that issue.

- *Smoking helps when stressed.* The feeling of stress is similar to withdrawal from nicotine, so by removing the symptoms of withdrawal your total feeling of stress is lessened (although nothing has been done to deal with the actual stressful situation).

- *Smoking helps to feel relaxed.* Again, nicotine withdrawal is similar in sensation to mild stress, so having a cigarette removes that sensation and allows you to feel relatively more relaxed (but is just getting you back to the baseline of a nonsmoker).

- *It is glamorous to smoke.* Despite the fact that smoking has become less commonplace and is harder to do in public places, it still seems to be associated with some level of hip indifference, rebellion, or relaxation. Personally, I don't think there's anything particularly rebellious or attractive about getting addicted to cigarettes to the point that it dictates your behavior and mood. And certainly there doesn't seem to be anything particularly sexy about having to take breaks at one of those rare locations where smoking is permitted. We need to change this impression of smoking being "cool" and replace it with the conscious truth that people smoke for the sole reason of appeasing their addiction—to avoid the feeling of withdrawal from nicotine.

Allen Carr's *Easy Way to Stop Smoking* is a great book that emphasizes the paradox in what smokers believe and hammers home the reality of the addiction. Plus it is written by a former smoker who inhaled sixty to 100 cigarettes a day before quitting.

And remember that the reason you want to quit smoking is to reach your own ultimate goal of being healthier. So again, I have a question for you reflecting back to your personal ignition statement (see page 40):

Why do you deserve to free yourself from your addiction to nicotine? What motivates you to escape from smoking, to save money, to live longer, and to feel better? Because . . .

Direct the Rider

The next step in optimizing your success for this most challenging of lifestyle changes is to direct the rider. You will need to set some clear goals and outline your initial steps in the "how" of the process. These actions, along with the additional suggestions for shaping the path (see below), work to increase your confidence in successfully achieving your goal.

This process could be as simple as coming to the realization that you don't need or want to smoke anymore then just stopping. This decision might be the end result of years of thinking about it and then having one health issue, one family member dealing with the consequences of smoking, one conversation with a health professional, one discussion with a former smoker—or one particular section of a book—tip you over the edge and release the hold smoking has on you.

If that is the case, it is certainly the simplest and most direct path to becoming a nonsmoker. For those who prefer to take that route, then I would wholeheartedly encourage you to read Allen Carr's book for further information, persuasion, and support.

I do need to make it clear, however, that this is not the same as quitting cold turkey or using the strength of willpower alone, which has only a 4 to 7 percent success rate. What I am talking about is *getting to the point where you truly believe that smoking is pointless and that you no longer feel that you need to smoke.* You are not giving anything up or depriving yourself but are excited to be free from nicotine. Again, as with any other long-term lifestyle modification, we are not equipped to suffer, so the goal is to be a happy nonsmoker and not a resentful and unhappy one.

As a physician, it doesn't really matter to me how people quit as long as they are successful at it. If the above method doesn't speak to you, then consider some other avenues to help you escape from your nicotine addiction.

Nicotine Replacement Therapy

With nicotine replacement therapy (NRT), you use a product (patches, gum, lozenges, sprays) to replace the nicotine you get from smoking with a safer, more manageable, and more controllable device. NRT can increase your chances of successfully quitting by 50 to 70 percent over using the cold turkey/willpower method, which brings the rate of success up to around 7 to 10 percent. NRT works to reduce the physical withdrawal from nicotine by providing it in a different form than in the cigarette. NRT also eliminates all of the other drugs, toxins, and chemicals in cigarettes that are a significant health issue; many of the risks of smoking seem to come from the combustion and burning of the cigarette itself.

The various NRT products available seem to be equally effective and can be used together if need be. For example, you could use the patch for the baseline nicotine delivery and then use the gum for any periodic cravings you have. NRT is safe to use for the vast majority of people and is thus provided over-the-counter.

Zyban or Wellbutrin (bupropion)

This drug is a prescribed medication that was originally, and still is, used to treat depression. It is not known how exactly it works for smoking cessation but has been found to be helpful in that regard, so the drug was remarketed that way. It seems to be as effective as nicotine replacement. Side effects include dry mouth, insomnia, nausea, and rarely (one in 1,000) seizures. Talk to your doctor to see if this avenue is appropriate for you.

Champix or Chantix (varenicline)

This drug helps to satisfy the nicotine receptors in the brain in order to decrease the physical craving for tobacco. The success rate with this drug appears to be two to three times that of using nothing and seems to be more effective than Zyban. The most common side effect is nausea, which tends to be mild to moderate and decreases with time. Once again, speak to your physician if you would like to consider this method.

E-cigarettes (e-cigs, vapes, or e-hookah)

This method of nicotine delivery involves the use of a device to heat up liquid containing nicotine and other chemicals into a vapor that is inhaled. The nicotine relieves the smoker's withdrawal symptoms and the delivery method mimics smoking, so it is understandably an attractive option for many people.

However, there are some concerning aspects. These liquids are not regulated by the US Food and Drug Administration and thus it is unclear what exactly the other chemicals in the liquids are. There is definitely a concern around potential dangers associated with them. It is also unclear if they actually help people quit smoking or get in the way of quitting. Some people end up with *more* nicotine in their system as they continue to smoke the same number of regular cigarettes and use the e-cigarettes in places that don't allow smoking. It may also be a gateway device to smoking for children, as some of these nicotine liquids come in a variety of candy-like flavors.

At present, there is better evidence and known safety around other forms of nicotine replacement, as well as other more effective ways to quit. Though the use of e-cigarettes is not currently recommended, it may still be a valid option for those motivated to truly quit smoking and use these items to *replace* their cigarettes.

Hypnosis, Acupuncture, Laser, and Other Treatments

There has been no evidence that these types of therapies are any more effective than quitting using willpower alone. However, they appear to be safe, so if you find one works for you, then I'm happy for you, as any route to becoming a nonsmoker is a good one.

Timing

It is often very helpful to pick a quit date that is meaningful for you. You may consider a date that has some importance, like your birthday. You might try to avoid any big events (weddings, Christmas) that you know will be stressful when you're going through the initial phases of quitting smoking. You may pick a time when you're away for work or on holiday to start this new routine away from your normal triggers.

But you also shouldn't delay quitting indefinitely as there is always some potential excuse on the calendar. If you are honest with yourself, you likely have no intention of continuing to smoke until the day you die, and it will be daunting whenever you plan on quitting—be it today, tomorrow, next week, or next year. Given that, you might as well circle a date on the calendar and free yourself from nicotine sooner rather than later.

Shape the Path

The final factor in our change model is to implement changes in the environment that make it easier for the rider on the elephant to navigate the path. In regards to quitting smoking, there are a number of ways to do this.

Know What to Expect

If you are ready to stop smoking, then you can increase your confidence by knowing what to expect as your body learns to live without nicotine. With any method of smoking cessation, there will be some element of withdrawal, so it is best to be prepared no matter your chosen method. When you stop smoking, you have to deal with two types of challenges—the *physical withdrawal* from nicotine and the *psychological* strain linked with the many behaviors, situations, and triggers associated with smoking.

The physical withdrawal is typically mild and is often compared to a hunger pang or a sense of emptiness. Most smokers already go through similar sensations anytime they have to go longer than an hour without a cigarette. I'm sure you can sleep through the night without having to wake up to smoke or you can sit through a movie, meeting, flight, or wedding without smoking. The challenge is to accept this mild discomfort and be happy that it is a sign of your body resisting the control nicotine has on it.

The nicotine levels start decreasing in your body right after you smoke your last cigarette and within three days there is no nicotine left. Therefore, these physical symptoms are typically gone by day three! I wouldn't be surprised if many of you have gone longer than three days without smoking in the past with no significant issue. You were physically through the withdrawal at that point; however, you were likely sucked back in by the psychological triggers of smoking.

These psychological feelings of withdrawal—which can feel very similar to the physical ones—are the most challenging aspect of quitting smoking. They typically settle down after three weeks but may crop up again anytime. You need to remind yourself of the victory you have already had over smoking and that "just one cigarette" can get you back to square one in terms of physical withdrawal. You also need to remember that there is no pleasure associated with the act of smoking itself, only the removal of a relatively mild source of displeasure (the withdrawal feeling).

Develop New Relationships

Let's face it: smoking has likely had a significant place in your life for a long time associated with comfort, relaxation, and stress relief. It has been your way of dealing with some of life's challenges and celebrating successes. So, in order to succeed as a nonsmoker, you may need to develop some new relationships to replace what you had.

Ideally, you may be able to realize that nothing needs to be replaced, because quitting smoking is a good thing and has not left a hole in your life. Replacing smoking with candy, sugarless gum, or chewing toothpicks may be initially useful but it also may prolong that impression that something is missing and keep the door open for a relapse. Consider substituting healthier ways overall to deal with stress and life's challenges: exercising more, connecting with friends and family, and eating healthier.

What about Weight Gain?

One note regarding potential weight gain when you quit smoking: eating more calories, not quitting smoking, causes weight gain. The feeling of withdrawal can mimic the feeling of hunger and some people eat as a response. Resist that urge and remind yourself that it is the nicotine still trying to control you. And even if you do gain a few pounds after quitting, the overall health benefits far outweigh that additional weight.

Use Tools and Support

The health consequences of smoking put a huge burden on health care in the United States and Canada. For this reason, there are many programs out there to help people quit smoking—take advantage of them.

You can access information, tips, tools, online support, regular follow-ups, and motivation via text message, as well as free telephone support. Smokefree and Smokers' Helpline are two free resources with lots of useful tools and support.

Don't Give Up on Giving Up

Becoming tobacco-free often takes multiple attempts. So, if you have a setback, that's okay. Try and try again.

If you end up having a cigarette, understand it as part of the process and don't let it derail your resolve to quit. Consider yourself an ex-smoker who had a small stumble rather than being hard on yourself and going back to your old habits completely.

While the rare person may succeed in quitting on their first try, for most it takes several attempts. Don't be dejected, but rather be compassionate to yourself. Quitting smoking is hard, so give yourself some credit and support during the process.

What about Marijuana?

Given the changing landscape, the proposed medical benefits of marijuana, and the legalization of marijuana in many jurisdictions, it is worth discussing some health aspects of this drug.

Healthy Lifestyle

First of all, no medical professional would ever suggest that using marijuana is linked to healthy living, improving outcomes, and decreasing risk of disease. Marijuana is *not* a supplement to take to improve your health and has the potential for significant negative side effects.

Medical Marijuana

Marijuana is a plant that contains multiple compounds with multiple effects on the human body that are not entirely clear. The proposed benefits of marijuana for medical issues are vast but largely *not* supported by evidence at this time.

PAIN MANAGEMENT

The most common use for medical marijuana is pain control, but the evidence is very weak and sparse. Some small studies show some benefit, but other non-opioid drugs have better evidence— and longer, larger, and better studies tend to show no benefit with marijuana.

One could argue that the risks of addiction and side effects with marijuana are less than with opioids or narcotics, so it may play a role as *part* of a chronic pain management strategy.

OTHER CONDITIONS

Proponents of marijuana usage often claim it has benefits for many other conditions, primarily anxiety, nausea, and spasticity. Evidence again is poor here and thus marijuana is not recommended as a routine therapy for these conditions either.

SIDE EFFECTS

Adverse effects of marijuana usage are common and probably underestimated given that people in studies tend to already be users, believe in the treatment, and it is impossible to blind the participants to who is and is not getting marijuana. Given that, studies show that one out of every eight to twenty patients will stop using the drug due to side effects. These range from low blood pressure to visual disturbance, hallucinations, or paranoia.

Overall, given the high risk of adverse effects and weak evidence for benefit, any trial of use for medical reasons should be considered very carefully. There are often other medications with better evidence to try first. But given the subjective nature of the typical goals of treatment with marijuana (relief of pain, nausea, anxiety, spasticity), there may still be a role for a small experimental trial on just one individual—yourself.

Recreational Use

Personally, I support the legalization and decriminalization of marijuana use for recreational purposes, with its associated taxation and regulation. People should be able to choose to use this drug, much like alcohol, and be confident in its content but also be aware of its risks. This does not mean I think it is safe nor do I recommend its use.

The biggest concern with marijuana usage is its effects on the developing brain. While the evidence is not clear, there are associations with decreased IQ, long-term changes in brain functioning, increased risk of schizophrenia, and other effects on social outcomes such as education, employment, chronic use, and use of other drugs. Despite the inconclusive nature of these findings, they are significant negative outcomes for a drug used for fun. There may be some controversy on what the legal age for marijuana use should be, but regardless teenagers should be educated about these risks.

Another factor is the uncertainty associated with marijuana and the metabolism of its psychoactive components. Due to the fat-soluble nature of cannabinoids, the drug can stay in one's body for a long time after one use (up to one month), and repeated use can cause a significant accumulation of the drug. Its effects also don't seem to be related solely to the level in the blood stream. Thus, it is hard to say how long the drug will affect the brain's overall functioning and its specific effects such as on driving ability and concentration.

On the positive side, we do know there are very few acute or sudden risks of marijuana toxicity, unlike opioids' risk of respiratory depression. We also see that marijuana doesn't seem as addictive as opioids or alcohol.

But chronic marijuana use disorder does occur and can affect motivation and one's future overall. We shall have to see if this becomes more prevalent with legalization.

My final thought in regards to the legalization of marijuana for recreational use is that I think adults should be free to obtain a safe product if they choose to partake in its *occasional* use and are aware of the risks and effects of the drug. I do have concerns about the potential for increased prevalence of chronic use and the risk for subtle and not-so-subtle effects on one's life.

Summary

If you are addicted to cigarettes, then quitting—or freeing yourself from—smoking is the best thing you can do for your health. As Allen Carr states, "You have nothing to lose and everything to gain."

The key aspect to successfully quitting smoking is finding your motivation—seeing and feeling the need to change. You can do this by realizing the perverse truth behind smoking: there is no pleasure or benefit associated with smoking beyond the temporary relief of the desire to smoke. In other words, the only reason to smoke is to briefly feel free of that urge to smoke and to allow the continued dependence on nicotine.

The benefits of quitting smoking include improving how you feel today and in the future (including the long-term freedom from that urge to smoke) and reducing the numerous health risks of smoking.

Once you truly feel that smoking is something you need to put behind you, you have numerous options to help optimize your chances of success. Quitting on your own is feasible if you see smoking for what it is and are confident that you can give it up. If not, you can look to resources available through government-supported smoking cessation programs, you can use over-the-counter nicotine replacement therapy, or you can consult your doctor for prescription drug support and for further information on options.

Having a life free of cigarettes is one of the most basic things you can do to improve your health. It is possible to do, as millions before you have already succeeded in that goal. You too can join that group—your first step is to make that commitment to try and to keep trying until you succeed.

8

Vaccinate

*"Vaccines are the most cost-effective health-care
interventions there are. A dollar spent on a
childhood vaccination not only helps save a life but greatly
reduces spending on future health care."*
Ezekiel Emanuel

THE TOPIC OF vaccinating our children has become very
delicate and difficult in the past few years. With parents
exposed to so much conflicting information on this subject, it is understandably very hard to know what to believe.
When you hear claims that vaccinations have the potential to
irreversibly harm your infant child—the most precious being
you could imagine—it is reasonable to be concerned and feel
apprehensive.

The responsibility one feels as a new parent adds weight
to every little decision: what kind of crib to get, to co-sleep or
not, what kind of car seat to buy, what kind of stroller to use,
to breastfeed or use formula, and which kind of formula to
choose? It is endless and can feel overwhelming, when all you
want to do is keep your little one safe and healthy. When it's

time for vaccination, you likely need more information to feel confident in your decision. The challenge is getting good information from someone you trust and feeling content enough with that information to take action.

The majority of people vaccinate themselves and their children, and a few people will never change their minds about the topic. This chapter is mainly directed at those who feel scared, confused, or want to feel confident in their decision. I hope that no matter where you land on this spectrum you will be open-minded enough to read this chapter in its entirety. I provide reliable information about one of the most successful health interventions humanity has ever developed, while clarifying some common myths about vaccination. I hope to convince you that vaccinations are a key aspect of healthy living for your family and yourself.

Any level of uncertainty around a difficult choice or a change typically leads to inaction. When it comes to vaccinating our children, it can be easier to delay indefinitely or avoid thinking about it, rather than commit to getting the immunizations done. But delaying or avoiding vaccinations puts your child—as well as the health of other children and people in your community—at risk. My goal is to help you feel confident enough in the recommendations of the global medical community to overcome any hesitancy and keep you and your loved ones up-to-date on your vaccinations.

I have joked that vaccination has become one of those subjects—like politics and religion—that are taboo to bring up in polite dinner conversation. The discussion of vaccination usually boils down to two views that cannot be reconciled. On social media, a post on anything related to vaccination programs seems to yield angry and visceral responses on both sides.

For this reason, I have been nervous to bring up this topic but I reassure myself by knowing I am in good company. I am thankful that prominent physicians, health writers, and community members—from Dr. David Gorski to Tara Haelle to Timothy Caulfield—have publicly expressed their support for vaccinations.

I truly am grateful for all those who have been vocal in this area, and they have helped me to be clear with my patients and friends about why I stand firmly on the side of vaccination. They have also motivated me to join the discussion and add my voice in support.

Why Vaccinate?

To begin, let's define the terms: *vaccination* refers to the use of a substance to induce an immune response that leads to immunization. *Immunization* is the process of becoming resistant to an infection, be it by surviving the illness *or* by vaccination. (I use both terms interchangeably in this chapter.) When we vaccinate someone, we are not giving them a "medicine" but tricking the body into producing its own antibodies, via a natural process, against the disease—without having to endure the symptoms, risks, and complications of the illness itself. It is a phenomenal process to prevent illness.

The bottom line when it comes to vaccines is that they are incredibly effective and safe. Medical practitioners, medical associations, public health departments, scientists, researchers, governments, and health organizations around the world all agree that vaccines are a good thing and should be provided to everyone *to protect and save as many lives as possible*. A debate implies that there is an ongoing discussion between opposing viewpoints; as far as the science is concerned, there is no "other side" on this subject. Some people, even a few physicians, disagree and believe there is a large conspiracy to try to harm our children; this group is a tiny minority. There are also tiny minorities who believe that the Earth is flat and only 6,000 years old, and that we didn't land on the moon.

Vaccines, and scientific findings in general, do not care if you believe in them or not. They help protect you no matter your stance.

In addition to the consensus among governments, health organizations, scientists, and physicians, it is important to note that the vast majority of people understand the benefit of vaccines. Despite the impression some patients have that there is true debate and controversy around vaccines, the reality is that worldwide about 85 percent of infants are vaccinated against polio, diphtheria, pertussis (whooping cough), and tetanus. In Canada, the results of a survey done in 2013 showed only 2.7 percent of children under age two had not received any vaccinations, while 89 percent had been vaccinated for measles, mumps, and rubella. In the United States, 2016 data from the Centers for Disease Control and Prevention show vaccination rates to be similarly high—92 percent of infants aged nineteen to thirty-five months were vaccinated for measles, mumps, rubella, and chicken pox.

My point is that the despite the vocal presence online, in the media, and at rallies, only a very small group is pushing an anti-vaccination agenda forward. Many of us in the medical community are frustrated when television "debates" present one person discussing the value of vaccination and another presenting the anti-vaccine point of view, in an attempt to fairly show both sides of the issue. This is a misrepresentation—to be accurate you would have to have dozens of people speaking to the value of immunization and one person trying to shout down the science.

Myth #1: There is controversy and debate around the safety and effectiveness of vaccinations.

Fact: Scientists, doctors, governments, and health organizations agree in the value of vaccination programs and their safety. The belief that they are unsafe or dangerous is held by only a very small group of people, as demonstrated by the high worldwide vaccination rates.

I do not mean to imply that we can be complacent. While vaccination rates are generally high, and the incidence of vaccine-preventable diseases has plummeted (polio and rubella are gone from the United States; diphtheria—which used to kill up to 15,000 Americans each year—is exceedingly rare), the rates of vaccination are dropping. They are also dangerously low in certain pockets of North America—for example, one school in California had 40 percent of students on some sort of exemption from vaccination, and another had only a third of students fully vaccinated—which can allow the reemergence of diseases that we have not seen for years.

This has already happened with outbreaks of measles. The outbreak in Disneyland in 2015 saw 159 people from eighteen states be infected and more than 80 percent of them were unvaccinated or did not know their status. In 2017, more than 20,000 people in Europe had measles, with thirty-five deaths. While there are multiple factors involved—low coverage in marginalized groups, challenges in vaccine supply or disease surveillance—the decreased uptake of vaccinations in traditionally safer countries has resulted in overall increased episodes throughout Europe.

In order to have an effective population vaccination program and protect our most vulnerable, we need to have an 85 percent vaccination rate for most diseases (like mumps and rubella); for the most contagious—like pertussis and measles—probably closer to 95 percent. We also have to be aware that even if diseases aren't common in North America, they are just a short plane ride away as seen with the measles cases in Europe. Even polio, which is almost eradicated around the world with a 99 percent drop in cases since 1988, still has cases reported in Pakistan, Afghanistan, and Nigeria. Travelers to and from these regions could still be exposed to the illness and bring it back to North America.

A common refrain from those against vaccination is that if your children are vaccinated and protected, then what do you care if others choose not to vaccinate. Well, beyond the fact that I think that all children should be protected and safe, the reality is that no vaccine is 100 percent effective—it depends on the immune system of the person as well. The most vulnerable of our population may not be able to get vaccinated with live vaccines and would not generate immunity with others, due to a weakened immune system from cancer, chemotherapy, medication, or another underlying disease.

It can be hard to think of that bigger vague picture of protecting others, so think of a real person. My mother-in-law had leukemia, chemotherapy, and an autologous bone marrow transplant: her immune system was weak and no vaccination would be useful to her. Instead, it was the responsibility of everyone around her to protect her—to reduce the risk of infection as much as humanly possible. Or think of the family of a child who is immune-compromised. How much fear must they have in sending their child to school, the park, or the mall knowing that any infection, let alone one of these vaccine-preventable ones, could send him to the hospital or even kill him.

Preventing outbreaks of these illnesses, even for those already vaccinated, comes down to the numbers. Vaccinated children are certainly better protected than unvaccinated ones during an outbreak, but again it is not 100 percent effective. When you look at the higher *proportion* of children who have been vaccinated, the *absolute numbers* who get infected may end up being larger among the vaccinated group. I know this is confusing, so let me use an example.

Let's say during an outbreak of a disease that the risk of infection in vaccinated children is only 4 percent and in unvaccinated children it is 40 percent. If 1,000 children are exposed and only twenty are unvaccinated, then eight unvaccinated children will get sick (40 percent of twenty). Thirty-nine children of the vaccinated group will get the illness (4 percent of 980). Some may use those absolute numbers to argue that vaccinations don't work, but clearly it is the opposite. We need high vaccination rates to stop the spread of the disease among all of our population—those vaccinated as well as those who can't be.

Myth #2: If you or your child is vaccinated, there is no reason to worry about whether other people are vaccinated.

Fact: The purpose of getting vaccinated is to protect you, your family, and your community at large. We need extremely high vaccination rates to prevent outbreaks of these diseases and protect everyone in our community, especially the most vulnerable who can't receive vaccines or for whom they are ineffective.

As vaccination rates drop below the threshold, we will likely continue to see outbreaks of these illnesses, and the potential is there for these diseases to once again become part of our medical landscape. We have been spoiled by the success of worldwide vaccination programs and forget about the potentially devastating consequences of these now vaccine-preventable diseases.

But we cannot allow complacency to put our children in harm's way again. Just because we don't remember these illnesses doesn't mean they don't exist. We need to be concerned with the reemergence of these illnesses because, at some point, children will start to die or have significant consequences from diseases like pertussis and measles—again as seen in Europe. It is a numbers game—as more people are infected, eventually someone will experience significant consequences. We even still minimize the risk of things like influenza—even though the flu vaccine isn't 100 percent effective, it is still one additional measure of defense against an illness that kills adults and children every year.

I don't want to use fear to push for vaccinations; I just want to emphasize how fortunate we are that vaccines have been so effective. We can't let this success blind us to how life used to be. It may be worthwhile to talk to seniors who have had more experience with these illnesses than most current physicians have had. Even polio is just a generation removed and celebrities like Alan Alda, Joni Mitchell, Neil Young, and Jack Nicklaus were all fortunate to have survived it.

Myth #3: These illnesses are rare, so I don't need to be worried about vaccinating for them.

Fact: Although rare, these vaccine-preventable illnesses are still around and have the potential to reemerge, particularly in our global community. It is up to all of us to ensure they don't.

I understand that it is very hard to change minds, but that doesn't mean it's not worth the effort. The anti-vaccination movement's narrative really appeals to the See-Feel-Change model we talked about previously. Seeing a parent express their belief that a vaccine caused irreparable damage to their lovely child, and seeing that same child in some state of distress really sticks in your mind. It causes all of us to *feel* something. Regardless of whether that anecdote is scientifically valid or not, the story is powerful.

The medical response tends to lean toward the Analyze-Think-Change model: a lot of data is presented that demonstrates that vaccines have been proven to be safe and effective, but that approach does little to overcome that narrative. The medical community's challenge has been to find a way to counter these strong emotional stories with compelling facts. It used to be that the numerous cases of children in hospital, quarantined, or otherwise affected by these illnesses was fresh in our minds and emphasized the importance of vaccination, but thankfully those incidents are few and far between. But I do wonder what the uptake would be for vaccines for more modern disease scares like the Zika virus or SARS—incredibly high, I suspect. I hope we can find other ways to demonstrate the value of immunization without going back to being fearful of illnesses killing or disabling our children.

Since the image of a healthy child with the absence of a disease is not that compelling, I will try to show you the common cognitive errors, logical fallacies, and biases involved in this issue. I'll return to the critical thinking concepts we discussed in the "Think" chapter. Realistically, the recommended *behavior* for this particular focus on healthy living—vaccination—is easy: book an appointment at your public health unit or with your primary care provider to update your children's and your own vaccinations. The true challenge is in the thinking: How can we feel confident in the information we have in order to move forward on that action?

Step 1: Focus on the Claim Itself

The first step in analyzing the issues around vaccination is to focus on the specific concern. Oftentimes, there is a general fear of "the shots" and it helps to clarify that. If the belief is that all vaccines are bad, then there is not much wiggle room. If there are absolutely no vaccines you would ever consider, under any circumstances, then it is unlikely that any information anyone could provide would ever change your mind. But hopefully there are specific concerns you have that I can help alleviate.

In focusing on the individual claims, it is again important to note that the *source* is not the target of the discussion. Any discussion descending to name-calling or personal attacks is not helpful. I will keep focused on the particular and common fears in an effort to reduce them.

One common worry is that vaccine programs begin at such a young age. Some parents are concerned that vaccinations can be harmful to their baby. The reason to vaccinate so early comes down to the basic philosophy of any vaccination program: *to ensure immunization occurs before the child has the chance to be exposed to the disease.* It does no good to give a vaccine at age two if the child is infected and suffers with it at age one. Vaccinations are given as soon as feasible to protect the child. In some cases, children are immunized shortly after birth to minimize the risk of transmission of an illness from mother to child (hepatitis B, for example). All of these vaccinations have been given for decades; after millions of doses being tracked and watched, the safety of this schedule is clear. For this reason, I do not advocate for any delayed immunization schedules—the concern is not founded and delaying makes children vulnerable.

Myth #4: Vaccines are given at too young of an age.

Fact: Vaccines are given as soon as possible to protect the child before any possible exposure to the disease.

Another concern parents have is that the immune system might become overloaded with all the shots that infants get as part of the vaccination program. Certainly, there have been more vaccinations added to the routine immunization schedule, and it can seem like a lot, but this is a good thing. The more illness and disease we can prevent, the safer our children are.

The reality is that our immune systems can handle it. Our immune system does not work based on the number of diseases it's exposed to but rather by the number of antigens—molecules that can induce an immune response. When exposed to a pathogen, like a virus or bacteria, the body creates antibodies to the wide variety and large number of antigens on it. With today's vaccinations, we are able to limit the number of antigens in the shots and thus the actual burden on our system is much smaller than if it was exposed to the whole virus. In fact, even with the increased number of vaccinations, our body is exposed to much fewer antigens than in earlier vaccination schedules. For this reason, I do not recommend an altered vaccination schedule that attempts to spread them out to decrease a risk that does not exist.

Myth #5: Our kids are given too many vaccines and it is too much of a burden on their immune systems.

Fact: Our immune system can handle it. In fact, the current vaccine schedule exposes the body to fewer antigens than used in the 1980s.

The next area of anxiety for many parents is that there are dangerous toxins in the vaccinations. With any substance, it is the dose that makes it dangerous or not; any substance will be toxic at high enough doses and anything given in a small enough amount will do us no harm. For example, you can die from drinking too much water and yet you will experience no appreciable effect from the small amount of opium in a poppy seed muffin. Typically, there are tiny doses of ingredients in a vaccine that serve to dissolve the antigen, stabilize it, or to create a more potent response to make it more effective, and these ingredients tend to be targeted by those in the anti-vaccine movement.

The initial concern raised was around mercury. This claim was focused on thimerosal, which is used as a preservative in some vaccines. Thimerosal is used presently only in the multidose flu vaccine and in one multidose version of the meningitis vaccine. It contains the mercury atom but breaks down to ethylmercury, which is vastly different from the methylmercury found in fish, which you have likely heard concerns about. Ethylmercury has been extensively studied since the initial concerns: it has been found to be quickly metabolized, much less dangerous than methylmercury, and harmless in the tiny doses used in vaccines.

Formaldehyde is another common toxin of concern. Formaldehyde is used to inactivate live viruses prior to vaccine production. There may still be tiny amounts remaining in the vaccine, but your body produces much more of it on its own. You are also exposed to it in many household items (nail polish, plywood, grocery bags), and you consume it regularly in fruits and vegetables.

Aluminum is also used in some vaccines to help make the immune response to the vaccine stronger. Again, it is in tiny amounts, and babies are exposed to much more through breast milk, formula, and their environment. Some vaccines may also contain tiny doses of antibiotics to prevent bacterial growth, and some vaccines may have trace amounts of egg protein remaining after the use of eggs to grow the viruses—neither of which is a concern.

And to dispel one other unfounded claim, there is no anti-freeze in vaccines.

Myth #6: There are dangerous toxins in vaccines.

Fact: There are tiny amounts of additives in vaccines to help make, store, and preserve the vaccine. Some components are there to help them work better. They are in tiny doses and have been repeatedly shown to be safe.

One of the most common and discussed fears around vaccinations is that they cause brain damage, autism, or other neurological issues. This impression has typically resulted from the spread of information, as follows: an initial report linking vaccination to brain injury is very publicly and vocally discussed in the media and online. Almost immediately vaccination rates decline. After the issue is analyzed and investigated by researchers, it is revealed to be unfounded, misleading, or totally false. However, this information is only quietly spread and never completely undoes the mistrust created by the initial report.

There are a couple of main examples of this. First, in the 1980s, a big concern was raised that the pertussis vaccine caused seizures and brain injury. As a result, congressional hearings were held and expensive investigations were ordered to determine the validity of the claim. An initial study did suggest a link and this terrified families and physicians alike. Unsurprisingly, the rates of vaccinations for pertussis declined dramatically. However, numerous repeat studies all over the world were never able to duplicate the findings of the initial review and consistently found no link between the vaccine and brain injury or seizures.

Finally, after detailed analysis, it was concluded that the *initial study was wrong.* Due to political pressure and to be sure that no one could accuse it of being biased toward proving the vaccine was safe, many cases were included in the investigation as potential examples of vaccine injury that were later found to be false—either due to other causes or the fact that the children were actually normal prior to and after the vaccine. Even more profound was the fact that Dr. Samuel Berkovic, a neurologist from Australia, was able to determine that many of these cases of supposed vaccine injury were due to Dravet syndrome, a genetic disorder characterized by seizures in the first year of life and subsequent developmental challenges. Unfortunately, all of this robust and detailed science that has ruled out the link between pertussis and brain injury has never quite removed that erroneous impression of risk around vaccines and brain development.

Considering vaccine risk, it is also worth noting that just a few reported cases of potential issues are enough to raise concern—when giving out millions of doses of vaccines, even a tiny serious risk is enough to warrant caution. This is a valuable approach to ensure a safe vaccine for the population. On the downside, a few errors in reporting can lead to unwanted anxiety.

Case in point is the issue around the measles, mumps, and rubella (MMR) vaccine and its purported link to autism. The initial paper by Andrew Wakefield, a British surgeon, was published in the respected medical journal *The Lancet* in 1998. It involved the report of only *eight* cases of autism that he linked to the MMR vaccine; again, this led to an immediate reduction in vaccination rates from which we are still trying to recover. We've experienced a drop in vaccination rates despite the fact that all subsequent trials have shown no link between vaccines and autism; that Dr. Wakefield's initial paper was retracted by *The Lancet*; that Dr. Wakefield was reprimanded by England's General Medical Council for not having his study approved by an ethics review board; and that Dr. Wakefield is now unable to practice medicine in England after being struck from the country's medical register.

The fact that one small study raising concern can galvanize the research community to determine the truth is encouraging;

the fact that one small erroneous paper can continue to create confusion and harm, despite the abundance of good evidence disputing it, is disappointing and worrisome.

Myth #7: Vaccines can cause autism, seizures, or brain damage.

Fact: Vaccines have been thoroughly investigated for safety against all of these claims and have been repeatedly found to be safe.

Step 2: Determine the Pre-test Probability

The next step in considering the safety and effectiveness of vaccines is the pre-test probability. In terms of vaccinations, that would be the likelihood that the entire medical community, pharmaceutical industry, governments, and health organizations the world over are all conspiring to give children vaccinations they don't need as a way to poison them and cause developmental problems.

I struggle with this one and try to not take it personally when this claim is made by patients or acquaintances. But it is a hard one to let go. As a family physician, I encourage my patients to be vaccinated and perform the vaccination; it's one of the core roles I have as a primary care provider. The idea that I would do this just for the money (and, for the record, vaccinating infants is not a high-paying endeavor) regardless of some significant potential harm it could cause patients is a bit insulting.

Setting aside my personal feelings, any conspiracy of this size would require the involvement of too many people to count, all keeping the truth a secret. How do we manage that? Where would the leadership meet? How does one benefit from this conspiracy to vaccinate children?

I don't want to belabor this point, as anyone who believes there is a conspiracy will likely believe that I am part of it as well. I just request that you honestly ask yourself: What is the likelihood of all of these parties—who in general don't work well together—being able to coordinate such a vast global conspiracy?

Myth #8: There is a complex conspiracy by government, health-care workers, and Big Pharma to poison our children with vaccines.

Fact: There isn't.

Step 3: Check for Biases

When looking at vaccine safety claims, even though the focus should be on the actual issue at hand, it is still worthwhile to consider where information is coming from and any potential biases or conflicts of interest. I understand that many people might think that, as a physician, I am unreliable to talk about vaccines because I'm part of the "system." I can somewhat see where that comes from but, again, I only get paid a few dollars for each vaccine given, and no amount of money would be enough to justify me putting children at risk. And in defense of the medical profession, and science in general, we are not held to a strict "belief" in vaccinations but rather to the evidence behind them; if that evidence changes, so do our practice and standards of care.

Changes in standards of care have already happened in numerous ways when it comes to vaccination. For example, a vaccine against rotavirus, a common virus that can hospitalize thousands of children each year in North America and kills thousands daily in the developing world, was released in 1998.

After ten months, some concerns were raised after reports of fifteen children apparently developing intussusception (a rare telescoping of the bowel, which is a medical emergency). Without any media pressure or scandalous revelation, the vaccine recommendation was removed and the product was pulled off the market until further studies were done. Eventually, a risk was found of one case in approximately 10,000 vaccine recipients, and it took seven years before a safer version was made and released for use.

That example shows science working to further our understanding and to ensure a safe vaccine program. If evidence is presented to change our body of knowledge, the medical community responds to it. In contrast, many in the anti-vaccine movement are held to a certainty bias that vaccines are harmful—they are sure they are right and nothing can be said or done to change that mindset. This makes any discussion on this topic very challenging.

Currently, the anti-vaccine campaign seems to be promoting the idea that they are all about access to information to allow parents to make their own choices. The name of the most powerful anti-vaccine organization in America, the National Vaccine Information Center (NVIC), makes this stance clear. Unfortunately, the name doesn't change what it does: provide misleading, inaccurate, and frightening information to parents in an attempt to discourage vaccination. The NVIC has consistently opposed any and all vaccinations—no vaccination appears to be safe enough or good enough for them to recommend. They are even against a vaccine that has been proven to prevent cancer—the HPV vaccine, which prevents cervical cancer.

I have struggled with this mindset, as I don't really understand how an intervention whose sole purpose is to prevent illness, complications, and death from disease could generate such mistrust and fury. I don't believe it comes down to financial motivation (although I'm sure there are many lawyers who make a good living representing these cases and that some doctors have done well as professional witnesses on the subject).

I wonder if this response stems from the incredibly intense feelings that must come with having a child diagnosed with a developmental issue, like autism. Believing that the vaccine they allowed to be injected into their child caused irreparable harm—*which is wrong and unfair to think*—could cause overwhelming guilt. If that is what they truly believe, then I suppose it is understandable to be consumed by such anger and blame. I am sorry for that because it is unnecessary to add that immense guilt to what must already be a very difficult situation.

Myth #9: The goal of those opposed to vaccination is to provide accurate information to families in order to allow them to make their own informed decisions.

Fact: The continued spread of false information despite accurate science is a danger to an effective vaccination program. These organizations have a bias against vaccinations and are working to undermine confidence in them. No vaccine will likely ever be safe enough or effective enough to warrant their approval.

We have already discussed one bias that is common amongst anti-vaccination advocates, the *certainty bias*, but the biggest one around this issue is that of *confirmation bias*—the tendency to look for, interpret, evaluate, and remember information in such a way as to confirm what we already believe. We may, for example, only read articles supporting our view of vaccinations' safety or danger, which unfortunately often also ridicules the opposing view. If you are fighting that urge and have continued reading this chapter despite feeling the discomfort that comes from being presented with an opposing view, I truly thank you—I appreciate the extra effort that takes.

As a family physician, I have the opportunity to try to see both sides regularly. Obviously, I want to ensure my patients and their children are vaccinated, so I look to the evidence behind that view. But I also care for those few patients I have who are against vaccinations or have serious misgivings. I don't dislike them; I want to genuinely help them and understand where they are coming from. For this reason, I look at what's on these anti-vaccination sites. At times, they can sound convincing and I feel anxious as they work to insert a bit of uncertainty about vaccinations. I can only imagine how hard it must be for parents trying to navigate this maze who don't know about the background, the typical tricks and subjects used, and the weight of evidence on the other side in support of vaccinations.

Some physicians have taken a strict line on this debate and elect to not take on any patients who will not vaccinate their children. I don't believe in that stance. My role is to be a trustworthy source to help clear up the confusion. I do not offer, recommend, or support any type of delayed or alternative schedules of vaccination, but I will give vaccinations to families whenever they are ready to receive them—and I make sure they know that I will bring up the subject every single visit.

It's also never too late to get vaccinated, so children can be caught up on their shots at any age. Even teenagers or young adults who have been unvaccinated as children have to get fully updated in order to apply for certain jobs (in health care, for example) or to travel to certain areas. It is also worth noting that adults are recommended to remain up-to-date with annual flu shots, the shingles vaccine, tetanus boosters, and other age-appropriate vaccinations.

Another bias that often comes up on the topic of vaccines is the idea that the government or doctors "can't tell me what to do." This subject is challenging; getting a needle does seem invasive, and is it really ethical to force people to get a vaccination if they don't want it? I struggle with this myself and certainly hope we don't ever get to the point that we have to force individual families to vaccinate in order to help protect the larger population. I just ask that you be aware of the internal resistance you may be feeling due to this issue and not make it a primary reason you are rejecting a vaccination.

Step 4: Assess the Basis of the Claim

Now we get to more specifics on the nature of the claims themselves. What is behind the idea that vaccines are unsafe, beyond what we have already discussed? There are a number of logical fallacies, or errors in thinking, that tend to drive this point of view, many of which we discussed in the first chapter, "Think."

The first to consider is the use of anecdotes as data. Many people have a specific story or incident that supports their belief that vaccines can harm children. But one story or even lots of anecdotes do not replace a scientific study. Numerous case reports have been used to suggest that vaccines are dangerous, but subsequent high-quality studies have proven them to be false. Certainly, those anecdotal incidents are likely more memorable, but we need to be strong enough to resist that aspect and focus on the accuracy of the science.

Myth #10: Recounting a story about vaccinations causing harm is equivalent to research.

Fact: The plural of anecdote is not data. Stories can be inaccurate in multiple ways and scientific research is required to truly assess the safety and risk of vaccinations.

Next is the idea that because one thing happened after another, the earlier event caused the latter. This issue is huge when discussing vaccinations because many developmental delays, seizures, autism, and other conditions of childhood start to show themselves and are diagnosed in the first year of life—just when children are getting most of their vaccinations. It is inevitable that some will start demonstrating symptoms close to the occasion of an immunization just due to timing. It can feel incredibly powerful and definitive to a family that one caused the other, but that is why we need to look at the evidence and the studies—to offset that emotional, and completely natural, assumption.

Myth #11: Because symptoms showed up after a vaccination, the vaccination caused the problem.

Fact: Many conditions are first noticed in early childhood and vaccination also occurs during that time. Correlation does not equal causation. Scientific research is required to clarify if one action truly leads to a particular event; its place on a timeline is not sufficient evidence.

The idea that anything natural is good and anything unnatural is bad is another common logical fallacy that shows up in regards to vaccinations. Some people seem to feel that it is better to get the measles or chicken pox, as we would develop stronger immunity that way. In some ways that may be true; if you endure and survive the infection, your body will have had a very robust immune response to every antigen on that virus or bacteria and will be well protected as a result. However, what also follows from this idea is that if you are unvaccinated against all of these diseases, and you don't get infected either, you will have weaker immunity than someone who is vaccinated. The vaccination triggers your immune system to go through its *natural* process of producing antibodies so it is already prepared to fend off future infections from that bug. And there is the added benefit of not having to get sick, not having to deal with a rash or other symptoms, and not taking the risk of getting complications or even dying from the infection.

Myth #12: It is better to get the infection itself than to get vaccinated.

Fact: It is best to be immunized and protected without getting infected at all, and thus avoid the risks of the disease.

If people believe that it is better to get infected rather than getting vaccinated to avoid the illness, they must on some level feel that it is no big deal to get sick in the first place. "We all used to just get the measles or chicken pox, and we all are fine." Many people did recover with no issues at all from measles, mumps, chicken pox, polio, and any of the vaccine-preventable diseases, but those who died from them or suffered significant consequences are not available to make their voices heard. We also tend to downplay the illness itself, the symptoms and discomfort caused by it, and the possibility of hospitalization even if there are no long-term consequences.

Myth #13: With some of these vaccine-preventable illnesses, the disease itself is no big deal, so why even worry about it?

Fact: We tend to underestimate the illness itself, and even a low risk of death or serious complications is something worth preventing.

Clearly there are a lot of arguments being promoted out there against the value and safety of vaccinations. It can be overwhelming and frustrating to try to defeat them all, as often it becomes a game of whack-a-mole—once you refute one claim, another one pops its head up. Hopefully, through critical thinking, you can understand the limitations of many of the statements against vaccinations and feel confident in addressing any other ideas you are presented with.

Facts about the Flu Vaccine

Every year there is concern and confusion around the vaccine for the flu. In addition to the myths discussed in this chapter, there are a few specific concerns around this particular vaccine that need to be addressed.

- We have to admit that the flu vaccine is not our best vaccine. Due to the changes in the influenza virus every year, the vaccine has to be developed each and every year to try to match the virus and be most effective. Each year, three (or four) strains are picked as the most likely to circulate that winter. Some years, the match is very close; other years, it is not as close as we'd like. This results in the flu vaccine being able to reduce your risk of getting sick by approximately 50 percent (somewhere between 30 to 70 percent depending on the year). This is still significant; I'm sure people would be open to interventions that reduce the risk of car accidents by that amount.

- We have to admit that most people do not get the flu. You are far more likely to get colds and other viruses than the flu. But if you do get the flu, it is no fun and you will be laid up for seven to ten days with fever, muscles aches and pains, and generally feeling lousy. And there is a small chance of you getting seriously ill, being hospitalized or even dying.

- This risk of complications from the flu is much higher for those who are elderly, very young, or otherwise immune-compromised. Unfortunately, the flu shot is the least effective for these groups due to their weaker immune system. If you want to help protect your grandparents, it is probably better that you and those around them get vaccinated (although your grandparents should also get the shot to at least get some protection).

- It is still possible to develop complications from the flu if you are otherwise healthy. It is a serious illness that results in hundreds of thousands of hospital admissions each year (an estimated 310,000 Americans in 2015–16) and the deaths of about 23,600 people in the United States each year. In children, 80 percent of the deaths are in the unvaccinated.

- You should get the flu vaccine every year, as each year the vaccine is a little different and protects against different strains.

- You cannot get sick from the flu vaccine. There is nothing living in it (or it's a highly weakened form of the flu—depending on the vaccine). People tend to get sick around that time because the shot is given out during the fall when common colds start making an appearance, or you were exposed to the flu before receiving your shot.

- The flu vaccine is safe for pregnant women and for children older than six months.

- The stomach flu is not the same as influenza. The flu shot does nothing to prevent diarrhea. It also does not protect against the common cold.

- Just because you've never had the flu, that does not mean you can't get it in the future. If you got the flu shot in the past and got the flu anyway, it doesn't mean the shot can't help you the next time. The flu vaccination reduces your risk of getting sick but doesn't guarantee you won't get the flu, though it likely would make your illness less severe.

- The flu shot is extremely safe. The risk of any significant complication has been shown to be miniscule with millions of doses given each year, and that tiny risk is far less than the risk of complications from influenza itself.

Overall, the flu shot is effective, safe, and can help protect the most vulnerable in our population each year. Please consider it.

Summary

Vaccination programs around the world have saved millions of lives and led to the eradication of smallpox globally, as well as polio in all but three countries. Previously common diseases that used to infect, hospitalize, harm, and kill our children are now so rare that it is hard for us to feel any sort of concern surrounding them. However, as vaccination rates decrease, the likelihood of these diseases reemerging and hurting our children is increasing, as seen by recent outbreaks of measles, mumps, and pertussis in North America and Europe.

Vaccines have been repeatedly shown to be safe and effective. Worldwide, millions upon millions of doses have been given, studied, and shown to be safe. There is no debate between scientists, physicians, researchers, or governments on this issue. The idea of there being uncertainty around vaccinations has been promoted by a small minority who are, simply put, in the wrong.

It is absolutely understandable that some families are uncertain or hesitant given this environment. While there are likely complicated reasons why there is so much anger and animosity toward the vaccination and protection of our children, the myths and reasons given for the hesitancy are able to be refuted both by evidence and by critical thinking. I hope that with some careful consideration, thought, and discussion with your trusted primary care provider, you can come to the same realization that the vast majority of citizens have reached—that vaccines are safe and that they work to protect the health of ourselves, our families, and the most vulnerable in our communities.

9

Screen

*"One way to become sick is to
start looking for something to be wrong."*
H. Gilbert Welch, MD, MPH

U P TO THIS point, I have been discussing ways to improve your health by focusing on how to change your behavior. I have also addressed some specific ways to improve how you feel now, as well as how to prevent or reduce the risk of disease in the future. The next best thing to prevention is to detect an illness before it has a chance to cause symptoms. Screening programs aim to do just that: pick up a disease process before you are even aware of it in order to treat it faster, earlier, and more effectively.

While it may seem like it should be possible to test for every disease imaginable, in reality there are not many conditions that can be appropriately screened for. Screening refers to testing large numbers of people (on a population level) who have no symptoms at all for a specific condition. In order for the screening program to be successful, some basic criteria need to be met:

* *The disease needs to be fairly common.* It is not feasible to test millions of people to try to find a few rare cases.

* *The disease must be significant enough to cause harm.* It doesn't make sense to screen populations for the common cold.

* *The disease must have an effective treatment available.* There is no point in diagnosing a disease early if nothing can be done with the information.

* *The early treatment of the disease must be more effective than treating it after symptoms appear.* There is no benefit to screening for pneumonia, for example, since treatment is as effective once it's clinically obvious.

* *There must be some sort of lag time in the disease.* If the disease progresses quickly, there isn't enough time between when the disease starts and when symptoms develop to make a screening program work—unless we screen on a weekly or daily basis, which is neither practical nor recommended for anyone.

As you can see, the criteria are specific and limit the number of diseases that can benefit from screening programs. We must also acknowledge that the majority of us will not actually get the condition being screened for (be it cancer, early heart disease, osteoporosis, diabetes) and therefore the majority of us will get no benefit from screening.

This may sound hard to believe given how prevalent these diseases seem to be, but the reality is that the risk of dying from common cancers and conditions is relatively small. For example, the risk of a sixty-year-old American woman dying of breast cancer in the next ten years is about nine out of 1,000, or 0.9 percent. (Alternatively, the likelihood of her *not* dying from breast cancer is 99.1 percent.) The risk of a seventy-year-old American dying of colon cancer in the next ten years is about fifteen out of 1000, or 1.5 percent (or of *not* dying is 98.5 percent). We very clearly remember the unfortunate cases of cancer in the media, community, and in our families and that tends to inflate our perceived risk.

I am not saying that screening programs are not valuable. Screening can be highly effective in picking up cases of certain conditions early, targeting higher risk individuals, and saving lives. I am suggesting that it is important to consider the potential harms of screening, as well as the benefits, and then decide if it makes sense for you.

The value of screening is likely oversold—with all of the breast cancer and prostate cancer awareness programs, for example—while the value of the truly preventive measures outlined in the previous eight chapters is not given nearly enough attention. There are a number of reasons, on both patient and physician sides. For the patient, it is easier to get a test done than it is to make the behavioral changes that can make a significant impact on your health; passive behaviors are always easier than active ones. For example, periodically getting your blood work done to check cholesterol or sugars is much simpler than making the daily dietary or activity changes that will actually lower your risk of a heart attack.

Similarly, for the physician, it is easier to order a test than it is to have a discussion to help motivate behavioral change. For health administrators as well, it is much easier to track the percentage of patients who have undergone certain cancer screening than it is to track quality lifestyle management counseling. Again, this is not to say that screening isn't important, but I want to acknowledge that it is easier to focus on screening than on the specific actions that can make much more of a difference to your health.

Before we get further into some of the details around screening, I need to be clear that this information does not relate to the process of investigating someone who has symptoms. That individual needs to be diagnosed—and that is a very different population from the asymptomatic people involved in screening programs. If you have symptoms, you should be assessed by your physician or primary care provider. Sometimes, an office visit where you discuss your symptoms and are examined will be enough to determine the issue; other times, more testing may be required and the criteria for that will be different than that of a screening test for someone who feels fine. *The bottom line is that if you are feeling something unusual, it is best that you get assessed by a health professional.*

Absolute Risk, Relative Risk, and Number Needed to Treat

Statistics needs to be addressed when talking about health, screening, and potential benefit. Don't worry, we won't get too detailed, but it is worth understanding the difference between the concepts of *absolute risk reduction* (ARR) and *relative risk reduction* (RRR).

The absolute risk reduction is a basic concept in that it tells us how much our risk is reduced by any treatment or intervention. Let's say that 10 percent of all people who have heart attacks and are not treated will die. That means that out of 100 people, ten will die without treatment, but ninety will survive. Now let's say that there is a new drug that will reduce that risk to 8 percent, so only eight people out of that 100 will die. This is an absolute risk reduction of 2 percent (10 - 8 = 2), so two fewer people out of 100 will die thanks to the medication. By taking the drug, you can reduce your risk by 2 percent. This also means that ninety-eight people wouldn't get any benefit from the drug: ninety will survive with or without it, and eight will die with or without it.

Since your risk reduced by 2 percent out of a baseline risk of 10 percent, your *relative risk reduction* is 20 percent (since two is 20 percent of ten). This would be meaningful if you knew that you were one of those ten people originally destined to die from the heart attack—but, of course, we can't know which group you are in, so that number is misleading. The RRR is often used to make a small absolute risk reduction (2 percent in this example) seem much more impressive (20 percent relative risk reduction) to elevate the perceived benefits of a treatment or drug.

In other conditions, your risk of dying may be incredibly low (say 0.01 percent) but the treatment may be able to reduce that risk by 50 percent (RRR), which sounds very impressive. But the absolute risk reduction is not nearly as exciting since your actual risk would only be reduced by 0.005 percent (ARR). For this reason, it is always best to consider the *absolute risk reduction* when discussing or considering interventions as it is more concrete and easier to understand and can better help you weigh the benefits of any treatments.

Another way to discuss those same numbers is with something called the *number needed to treat* (NNT). This is determined by dividing 100 by the *absolute risk reduction*, which in our example gives us fifty (100/2). It means that you would have to treat fifty people with this new drug to save one life. The NNT is another tangible concept to use when determining the value of treatments, screens, and medications to an individual.

If you are expecting certainty with any test or treatment, then unfortunately you are expecting more than they can provide. Uncertainty is the norm when it comes to the potential benefits and harms of medical interventions. But becoming comfortable with these concepts and terminology is very useful and will help you make personal decisions around health. Understanding the limits of these tests may put more responsibility on your own behaviors but may allow you to feel less stress about the role of testing in your life.

Potential Benefits of Screening

As a public health intervention, screening—picking up a disease earlier before it has a chance to cause harm, grow, advance, or spread—makes perfect sense. Today, we have many ways to image the body with X-rays, ultrasounds, angiograms, CT scans, MRIs, and PET scans. We have ways to test less invasively than ever before with blood tests, genetic tests, and stress tests, as well as less invasive biopsies for samples of tissue.

We thus have ample opportunities to test and screen to find diseases earlier. As stated above, if the disease meets the criteria to warrant population screening and the test is appropriate, then *screening can save lives*. That is the ultimate benefit. And what's the harm of more information when compared to that? Well, that is the challenge—there is potential harm from testing and it tends to get underplayed compared to the promise of early detection and peace of mind. So, what are the actual risks of more testing?

Potential Harms of Screening

False Positives and False Negatives

It is important to be aware of the limitations of tests and screens. No test is 100 percent accurate, particularly when it comes to screening tests. There will be false positives and false negatives. (In medicine, a negative test result is typically a good thing—it means that you don't have the disease. A positive test suggests that you have what was tested for, so it's usually unwelcome).

A *false positive* is when the test is read as positive but the individual does not actually have the disease. A *false negative* is the opposite: the test is negative but the individual actually does have the condition.

	Positive Test Result	Negative Test Result
Person has condition	true positive	false negative
Person does not have condition	false positive	true negative

Screening tests tend to have a very low false negative rate; we do not want to say people don't have cancer if they actually do. This is not to say that screening tests don't miss things, but it is very hard to prove as a missed diagnosis could be due to a rapidly growing cancer. The result of erring on the side of caution is a significant number of positive results that go on for further testing and eventually come back negative—a false positive.

False positives are one of the biggest concerns with screening because they can cause significant harm. First, the anxiety that comes with a positive screening test and the potential diagnosis of cancer is emotionally difficult for patients. Even if the results eventually come back as negative, the experience can be very traumatic.

Second, further testing can be worrisome and never-ending. Subsequent tests can often lead to a biopsy, which involves some sort of procedure to get a sample of tissue to be analyzed. A biopsy has its own risk of infection or other complications depending on the type of procedure required.

And the more tests that are done, the more likely it is that an individual will have a false positive test result. For example, if a specific screening test has a false positive rate of 3 percent, and you have it done every year for ten years, then there is a more than 25 percent chance of you having a false positive test result at some point. Combine that with other tests being done, and the risk of having a false positive is even higher.

The challenge is determining how best to manage these risks with the benefits of screening. Public health and screening officials try to balance the number of tests, the kind of tests, and the frequency of tests to justify the number of false positives and minimize the number of cancers missed. It is something for you to consider when deciding what it is best for you.

Over-diagnosis and Over-treatment

Another risk of any screening program is the possibility that someone will be labeled with a disease or diagnosis but nothing is gained in that it doesn't change our recommendations. For example, a diagnosis of pre-hypertension (blood pressure in the borderline range) or pre-diabetes (elevated sugar but not enough to be called diabetes) may not be treated by your doctor beyond an emphasis on the need for eating better and exercising more—which should be highlighted for everyone regardless of any particular pre-diagnosis.

These types of labels have the potential to compel patients to focus on the fundamental aspects of good health, but such a pre-diagnosis may also lead the physician and patient to feel anxious enough to use medication that they otherwise wouldn't. And these medications might have significant risks and side effects, with minimal benefit to patients' health.

In terms of cancer, it can be a challenge to tell the difference between cancers that you are more likely to *die with* versus ones you would *die from*. This uncertainty can be hard to bear, so most patients (and physicians) tend to err toward more tests, more biopsies, and more aggressive treatments, like chemotherapy. Unfortunately, it's very difficult to know if a patient benefited from that treatment or not.

Lead-time Bias

It often seems that screening and early treatments help improve outcomes when looking at the five-year survival rates for particular cancers and treatments. The survival rate is the percentage of patients with a disease who will still be alive five years after diagnosis. For example, for bladder cancer the rate is 78 percent which means that of 100 people with bladder cancer, seventy-eight would be living five years after diagnosis.

This type of reporting can be misleading, however, due to *lead-time bias*. This bias suggests that any apparent improvement in survival is only due to early diagnosis; there is no change in the actual course of the illness. Imagine that you are standing on railroad tracks with a train (cancer) heading toward you. With a lead-time bias, the improved survival rate is due to seeing the train sooner rather than actually slowing it down.

Incidental-omas

Whenever you do a number of tests or screens, there is always the risk of discovering something unexpected. For example, doing a full-body MRI or CT scan often leads to the discovery of cysts or lesions on the liver or kidney. Now that they are seen, these lesions cause understandable anxiety, often have to be worked up, and usually lead to more imaging and maybe even a biopsy. It is very rare for these to be diagnosed as anything meaningful, but once something like that is seen, it does need to be evaluated.

This is a common consequence of having tests done "just in case" or "just to be sure." As a physician, I often feel annoyed with myself for ordering a test I was on the fence about and then finding one of these incidental-omas which the patient and I now have to deal with. Sometimes even if repeat imaging shows no growth and no worrisome features, the patient still elects to have it removed surgically or dealt with more aggressively, simply because they know it's there.

False Sense of Security

Patients may not be aware of the limitations of what tests can rule out. Getting normal results on a test may give you a false sense of security. A common example is doing an ECG or heart tracing in someone with no chest pain: a normal result may give you the impression that you don't have heart disease and aren't at risk of a heart attack. But the real purpose of the test is to look at the rate and rhythm of your heart, determine if you have had a previous heart attack, or see if your heart is enlarged due to high blood pressure. It doesn't tell us what your risk of future heart attacks might be. Another example is when patients are told their cholesterol is "normal." This result can lead you to think, "My doctor says I'm doing fine, so I can continue eating and (not) exercising as I have been!" That is not the intent of those kinds of tests: eating better and exercising more will *always* be a good idea to reduce your risk—regardless of the test result.

Misdirected Energy

Screening tests are a fairly black-and-white health intervention, which has appeal for physicians, health authorities, and patients alike. For the health practitioner, the test is either done or it isn't, and rates of completion can fairly easily be tracked. For the patient, it is easier to have these tests done than to make significant lifestyle modifications. You can see how more time and resources are drawn to screening and less to the more challenging work of changing behaviors around diet, exercise, sleep, and all the other subjects discussed in this book.

In addition to these screening recommendations personally taking my focus away from these important lifestyle issues, they can also prevent me from addressing my patients' specific concerns about their health. In effect, we may have competing agendas—I am trying to find time to ensure that all the recommended screening is done, as well as target any higher risk behaviors that can be improved, and you may have a list of entirely separate concerns you would like discussed. This makes it even more difficult to address everything in a short office appointment and may affect our relationship and sense of satisfaction with the consultation.

Choosing Wisely: Test and Treat Appropriately

While I have outlined potential concerns around screening, many of these issues apply to over-testing and treating in general. If you have a symptom, the criteria are different for tests, but the concerns are the same. You should be seen by a health professional to determine your risk and receive a likely diagnosis; still you should understand that additional testing has similar risks, as discussed. Your physician can determine the likelihood of any concern (your pre-test probability), which helps you decide if any test or treatment adds further value. Getting more tests or interventions isn't always better—for the reasons outlined in this chapter.

This is the basis of the Choosing Wisely campaign (ChoosingWisely.org), which helps clinicians and patients engage in conversations about unnecessary tests and treatments and make smart and effective care choices.

Screening Is Still Important

Despite all that I've written so far in this section, I am not against screening—it serves an important role in primary care, public health, and the prevention of significant disease. Screening large populations of asymptomatic people can result in lives saved. Given that, as well as the cost benefit of treating these conditions earlier, the risks of false positives and other potential downfalls may well be worth it. I just want to make sure you are aware of the factors to consider when choosing to be screened.

Different jurisdictions may receive slightly different recommendations for the same disease and screening test. The main organizations I reference here are the US Preventive Services Task Force (USPSTF) and the Canadian Task Force on Preventive Health Care (CTFPHC), which develop clinical practice guidelines for providers to deliver preventive health care. Since individual judgment varies, it may be a perfectly reasonable choice for some patients to choose not to undergo any particular test, despite the recommendations of the task force.

In the next section, we will look at the current recommendations for specific screening interventions to help you make your own informed choices. Keep in mind that recommendations are adjusted from time to time and further discussion with your health care provider may well be warranted.

Common Screening Tests and Interventions

Periodic Health Examination

The annual physical exam has been a mainstay of primary care from the beginning and many patients still believe they should come in annually for a check-up. The evidence suggests that this is not necessary, and most primary care organizations are moving toward recommending something called a periodic health examination (PHE).

The PHE is subtly different from an annual check-up and I like to think of it as a *check-in* rather than a *check-up*. The idea is to be assessed periodically to update family history, review any modifiable risk factors (smoking, diet, exercise, sleep, alcohol), screen for any concerning symptoms, and evaluate the need for any screening tests or vaccinations. Some of these assessments and reviews can be done during an appointment for other minor complaints to make more efficient use of time. Depending on the results of that review, you may require some blood work, other tests, and annual follow-ups. The difference from the old annual check-up is that the interval between exams is not based on the calendar but on the needs of the individual.

During these assessments, a complete physical examination is often not required as there is very little benefit from my examining an asymptomatic individual from head to toe; the likelihood of me finding anything meaningful is exceedingly low. Performing a specific examination really depends on the discussion and on any patient concerns. Certainly, height, weight, and blood pressure are reasonable measures to obtain at these times.

I have concerns about the value of "executive health physicals" where higher-level executives, or people willing to pay extra, obtain annual check-ups with additional tests (ECG, prostate checks, bone density, body fat composition, full blood work panel) that are not supported by evidence. These extensive physicals can give the impression that a regular health assessment isn't good enough and more testing is better, implying that the patients' own providers aren't ordering tests because we are cutting costs or are not being thorough. In actuality, the tests are not offered because there is no evidence of benefit, they offer a false sense of security, and they may cause harm. I recall talking to a thirty-five-year-old male who felt he got better care because he had a prostate exam during one of these executive physicals. I was reluctant to tell him that he had received a rectal exam for no rational reason whatsoever.

Overall, it is important to check in with your physician periodically to review any risks and concerns and to see if you are due for any routine screens and vaccinations. Beyond that, focus on the things you can do every day to be healthy—eat well, move, sleep, and enjoy your life.

Health assessments to review risks and symptoms and to determine whether any testing, screening, or vaccinations are required should be done periodically—consider two times in your twenties, three times in your thirties, three to four times in your forties, and every one to two years from fifty onwards. Frequency of assessment may change based on the individual's health needs.

Breast Cancer Screening

Breast cancer is one of the most common cancers we hear of and one that strikes fear in families everywhere. While screening is very important, we need to be honest about the risks, benefits, and limitations of mammograms, a radiological test used to pick up changes in the breast tissue. Both the USPSTF and the CTFPHC recommend women aged fifty to seventy-four undergo mammograms every two years. There is some evidence that mammograms provide at least a moderate benefit, but it is certainly not clear. The CTFPHC provides a number needed to screen of 720 for women aged fifty to sixty-nine in order to save one life; this would also result in twenty-six unnecessary breast biopsies and 204 false positive mammograms. Any individual would be reasonable to weigh their level of concern around breast cancer against their willingness to risk a false positive and a biopsy.

In regards to younger women aged forty to forty-nine, the evidence is less positive; the CTFPHC does not recommend screening in this group. Breast cancer is rarer and women's breasts tend to be denser in this age range, thus making it harder to see any significant changes in the mammograms. (Annual screening is recommended if a woman chooses to pursue screening in her forties.) We also have to acknowledge that cancers in younger women may be a different beast than that seen in older women, often growing faster or harder to detect. The USPSTF recommendation is a bit subtler for women in their forties: it suggests discussing the pros and cons to decide. The number needed to screen in this age group is higher with 2,100 women needing to be screened to save one life, again resulting in seventy-five women having unnecessary breast biopsies and 690 having a false positive mammogram.

So, while breast cancer screening is routinely recommended, determine what feels right for you and have a further discussion with your physician if so desired. It should also be noted that the evidence for screening is focused on mammography; other modalities such as ultrasound and thermography (infrared) are not recommended. MRIs may have a role in screening those with significantly higher risk (known carriers of breast cancer genes, very strong family history, for example) but is not recommended for the average population.

Mammograms are recommended every two years for women aged fifty to seventy-four. Testing for those women aged forty to forty-nine and for women older than seventy-four should be discussed with a primary care provider.

Colorectal Cancer Screening

Colorectal cancer (CRC) is particularly well suited for screening. Most of these cancers seem to progress linearly from a small polyp in the large bowels to a full-blown cancer slowly over ten to twenty years, and there is a long asymptomatic phase in which it can be detected. Unfortunately, the process of screening for this type of cancer involves handling poop or having a camera inserted up the rear end, which leads to low screening rates. We definitely have room for improvement with this screening program.

The main choices for screening for CRC are a stool test that looks for microscopic blood (fecal occult blood testing, or FOBT) or hemoglobin (fecal immunochemical test, or FIT) and direct visualization with a sigmoidoscopy or colonoscopy. The sigmoidoscopy examines the lower portion of the large intestine, the sigmoid area where most cancers are found, whereas the colonoscopy looks at the whole thing. There is a higher risk of complication (bleeding or perforation) the further along you go.

Given the poor uptake on testing, really any test you are willing to do is acceptable. The best idea is to talk to your physician about screening options, overcome any embarrassment, and pick the one that you would be willing to do.

Colorectal cancer screening via stool tests or sigmoidoscopy/ colonoscopy is recommended for all individuals aged fifty to seventy-four. Patients with normal results can repeat the stool tests every two years and direct visualization every ten years.

Cervical Cancer Screening

The Papanicolaou test, or Pap test, has been used successfully for years to detect the pre-cancerous changes that can eventually lead to cervical cancer. We know that these changes are triggered by the human papilloma virus (HPV) and are now largely preventable with the HPV vaccines. However, as there are multiple strains of HPV and the vaccines do not prevent them all, Pap tests are still recommended even if you have had the vaccination. Also, since HPV is associated with sexual activity, Pap tests are recommended when women are twenty-one years old or whenever they become sexually active—whichever comes *later*.

In the US and Canada, it had been common for women to be recommended annual Pap tests and screening for sexually transmitted infections (STIs). The current guidelines suggest testing much less frequently—once every three years—and this change has created some anxiety for women who fear it is too long a gap. Evidence does support this change, however, and other countries have gone this route far in advance of us. The Netherlands tests every five years and they do not have any higher rates of cervical cancer in comparison.

Also, be reassured that STI screening can still be done very effectively with urine and blood work as desired. And please be more reassured that pelvic exams or bimanual exams (where the uterus and ovaries are palpated internally) are *not* recommended for the routine check-up of women with no symptoms.

Cervical cancer screening via the Pap test is recommended for all women who have been sexually active and is to be done every three years between the ages of twenty-one and sixty-nine.

Prostate Cancer Screening

No screening test is the subject of as much confusion as the prostate specific antigen (PSA) blood test for prostate cancer in men. It used to be recommended routinely for men as young as age forty to help detect and treat prostate cancer early. Those recommendations have now changed and both the USPSTF and CTFPHC have recommended against using the test entirely; however, the American group has recently updated their guidelines to recommend that men aged fifty-five to sixty-nine discuss the pros and cons with their physician. The American Urological Association has agreed with that age group, while the Canadian Urological Association recommends starting the discussion at age fifty; both associations have emphasized the need for shared decision-making to allow the patient to decide what they want to do. No group is offering a clear recommendation for the test at this time.

Why is there so much concern around the PSA test? After all, it's a noninvasive blood test that simply provides more information. Well, it is likely the best example of many of the potential harms caused by unnecessary screening. First, most men will develop some element of prostate cancer as they age, so if we look for it, there is a reasonable chance of finding it. But most prostate cancer is slow-growing and something men will *die with* rather than *die from*. The challenge is determining who will develop the more aggressive forms of prostate cancer that we really want to catch early.

In addition, there is a high false positive rate on the PSA test. A high level could indicate many things beyond prostate cancer: infection, irritation, inflammation, or even inconsistency in the test results themselves. The follow-up tests required to work up any elevation of the PSA are invasive and have high complication rates. Biopsy is done via transrectal ultrasound, and you can appreciate that the infection rate when doing a biopsy through the rectum is higher than many other places. Treatment of prostate cancer is also risky in that surgery and radiation can lead to common side effects, such as impotence and incontinence, which greatly affect quality of life.

When you look at the numbers needed to screen, studies tend to break it down as follows. For every 1,000 men screened for prostate cancer via the PSA test between the ages of fifty-five and sixty-nine, one man's life will be saved but thirty-three men will undergo treatment with no benefit whatsoever and with all the risks and side effects. Sixty-three more men would have developed some symptoms of their prostate cancer but would not have died from it regardless. Of course, of those treated, we cannot know which one life was saved and likely all of them will believe treatment saved them.

Clearly this is not a straight-forward decision to make. But the good news is that there is not a right or wrong choice—and there is no need to panic with a slightly elevated reading. The management of these tests is getting less aggressive as a result of the evidence; now a positive result may lead to a watchful, waiting approach rather than a rush for surgery. Hopefully further information in the coming years will provide more guidance to best screening practices for this disease. In the meantime, think about the numbers and discuss testing further with your physician.

Prostate cancer screening via the PSA blood test is not recommended routinely. Discussion and shared decision-making is reasonable for men aged fifty-five to sixty-nine and who have a greater than ten-year life expectancy. If screening is agreed upon, then testing every two years is appropriate.

Osteoporosis Screening

Another condition that is worth screening for is osteoporosis and the risk of a hip fracture. The bone mineral density (BMD) test looks at the amount of bone at your hip and spine with a specialized X-ray test; that result is compared to a standard outcome to give you a score. This score, along with other information such as your age, sex, weight, height, and presence of other risk factors (smoking, previous fractures, family history of hip fractures, use of steroids, alcohol usage, and other health conditions) is used to determine your risk of having a hip fracture in the next ten years.

If the calculation puts you in the low-risk category (0–10 percent risk of fracture), then nothing more needs to be done and a repeat BMD test and calculation should be done in five years. Those in the high-risk category (>20 percent) would be recommended to go on medication and the BMD could be repeated in two to three years. For those in the middle (10–20 percent risk), discuss the pros and cons of medication with your medical provider to decide. Regardless of your risk category, everyone benefits from the general principles for reducing fractures and improving bone health—such as exercising, ensuring you are getting adequate calcium and vitamin D, and reducing your risk of falls.

The big thing to note for osteoporosis screening is that we are determining risk of fracture. *We are not treating bone density.* Patients often want annual BMD tests while on medication or to "see how they are doing." That is not the purpose of the test or the medication. Most medications that target bone health help to improve the *strength* of the bone and not the amount, and this difference is not detected by the BMD test.

Fracture risk calculation and BMD testing should be offered to those sixty-five and over and to those who are at higher risk. Intervention and further testing frequency will be dependent on the results of the initial test.

Cardiovascular Risk Screening

One major non-cancer issue that is screened for is cardiovascular disease, or the risk of heart attacks and strokes. This is not really screening in the typical sense in that we are not trying to diagnose people before they develop symptoms; we are trying to identify people who are at higher risk earlier so we can intervene to modify risk factors. The terminology and methods we use make it sound like we are diagnosing and treating something more specifically, which can be confusing.

Cases in point: the ideas of high cholesterol and even high blood pressure (or hypertension). High blood pressure can cause symptoms if the blood pressure is sky-high but, far more commonly, people feel the same whether their blood pressure is high or normal. Similarly, people experience no difference in how they feel if their cholesterol is high or low.

We use these numbers to help determine the risk of having a heart attack or stroke, similar to how we determine the risk of people having a hip fracture. These values are plugged into a formula, which is based on studies done on large populations of people over long periods of time, to determine a risk score for an individual. Other factors included in this calculation include family history of heart attacks, smoking status, age, and sex.

These formulas aren't perfect, but they give us a place to start and guide the discussion. Once we determine your individual risk of a heart attack or stroke, then we can look at ways to reduce that risk by considering your *modifiable risk factors*, which include exercise, diet, weight, smoking status, alcohol intake, addition of cholesterol medications, and blood pressure control. These are opposed to *non-modifiable risk factors* like your age and sex (males are at higher risk).

Regardless of your level of risk, there is obvious value in making positive lifestyle changes to improve your health. By focusing on them first, you may be able to keep your blood pressure and overall cardiac risk low and avoid or delay the need for medications.

When blood pressure is an issue, we are not in fact "treating" your high blood pressure but rather aiming to lower your risk of a heart attack or stroke by lowering your blood pressure. Hypertension is a major modifiable risk factor for those events, so maintaining a healthy blood pressure is very important. For this reason, it is advised that all adults get their blood pressure checked during routine visits.

The general idea is that the lower the blood pressure, the better. But the actual targets differ depending on other factors such as the presence of diabetes or kidney failure. In most cases, the target for blood pressure is to be less than 140/90.

Maintaining a healthy weight, exercising regularly, decreasing salt intake, eating more fruits and vegetables, quitting smoking, and limiting alcohol consumption can all help in that regard. For a substantial number of people, that will not be enough to get their blood pressure to target, so medication is commonly required *in addition to the lifestyle changes.*

When it comes to cholesterol, the situation is more confusing. Although medications (statins, like Crestor and Lipitor, are the class of medication most commonly used and most studied) do lower cholesterol, the main benefit of them is to reduce your risk of a heart attack. Studies have shown that almost all statins reduce that risk by about 25 percent (relative risk reduction) at any dose but maybe up to 35 percent at higher doses.

By using your baseline cholesterol levels and calculating your overall heart disease risk, we can convert that relative risk reduction to an absolute one to help you decide if taking a statin makes sense for you. For those who are calculated to have a low risk of heart attacks (<10 percent), it is recommended to repeat a cholesterol test in five years and recalculate the risk. For moderate risk individuals (10–20 percent), consideration of therapy with statins is definitely warranted. For those at high risk (>20 percent), therapy should definitely be offered and preferably a more aggressive treatment. It should be noted that there may be different thresholds depending on the specific calculator used, the specific guidelines followed, and the decision-making process between the patient and physician.

By discussing your overall heart disease risk, instead of just your cholesterol levels, we can expand this conversation to address other ways to reduce your risk through lifestyle changes like stopping smoking, exercising more, limiting alcohol intake, losing weight, and improving your diet. From this standpoint, we're not "treating" your cholesterol; we're trying to reduce your heart disease risk, and there is no other effective test for that. If your risk level and your outlook lead you to take the medication and you tolerate it well, it is like taking a supplement with a large evidence base showing a relative risk reduction of 25 to 35 percent in regards to heart disease and stroke—that's far better than an aspirin a day or any other supplement out there.

Cholesterol Controversies

It should be noted that there is a lot of controversy around the role of statins and cholesterol levels in heart disease. Most cardiologists believe in the cholesterol model of heart disease and aim for lower and lower levels of cholesterol; others focus more on the overall heart disease risk and feel no studies have shown that treating to cholesterol targets has been clearly beneficial. My feeling, as a primary care physician, is that focusing on cholesterol specifically takes the focus away from the more practical and concrete idea of your overall heart disease risk. Taking a statin is simply one significant way to modify your risks—in addition to the other lifestyle modifications discussed

Screening for high blood pressure should be done periodically at routine visits, but at least following the same frequency as suggested for periodic health assessments. Screening for heart disease

risk using cholesterol values and a risk calculator should typically start at age forty for men and age fifty for women. Subsequent testing can be done every five years.

Diabetes Screening

Diabetes is a very common condition and associated with obesity, increased waist circumference, and the North American diet in general. Rates of adult-onset diabetes are increasing and we know that diabetes is associated with a higher risk of heart attack, stroke, kidney damage, retinal problems, and peripheral nerve issues. As a result, we try to detect it early so we can intervene early with a more aggressive approach to factors associated with these complications (lifestyle modifications, smoking, blood pressure, use of statins) in addition to improving sugar levels.

While routine screening is not recommended for those at low risk, I must admit that a check of sugar levels is commonly added to blood work. Ideally, it is best to use a validated risk calculator and/or target screening to those at higher risk (those with other cardiovascular risk factors, family history of diabetes, previous results showing high sugars, increased waist circumference, and those who are overweight or obese).

Routine screening for type 2, or adult-onset, diabetes should be offered to those at high risk of diabetes, as determined by direct assessment and/or a validated risk calculator. Repeat screening can be done every three to five years as deemed appropriate. Consideration of screening should begin at age forty.

Abdominal Aortic Aneurysm Screening

An abdominal aortic aneurysm (AAA) is a swelling or dilation of the main artery in your abdomen which, if enlarged, has a risk of spontaneously rupturing and bleeding—a catastrophic event with a high risk of death. If detected early, it can be treated surgically to greatly reduce this risk.

AAAs are thankfully not very common, but the risk is significantly higher for men, particularly for men who smoke. In terms of numbers needed to screen, in a group of 1,000 men—aged sixty-five to eighty, smoker or otherwise—one life will be saved and an additional two will avoid a non-lethal rupture. This gives us a number needed to screen of 1,000 men to save one life, but only 333 men to prevent a ruptured AAA. If limited to just male smokers, the number needed to screen to save one life is reduced to approximately 500.

Screening for AAA is recommended via a one-time ultrasound for men aged sixty-five to seventy-five who have ever smoked. In Canada, that recommendation is expanded to all men, smoker or otherwise, aged sixty-five to eighty. Follow-up is determined by the results of the initial ultrasound.

Other Conditions Not Listed Here

While we wish there could be effective screening programs for other diseases or cancers, the reality is that there is currently no effective way to do it for various reasons:

- A cancer may be too rare to warrant population screening.

- A cancer may progress or spread too quickly to pick up in the asymptomatic phase.

- We just don't have an effective test for that particular condition.

Common conditions where we hear tragic stories and wish there was something to be done include ovarian cancer, pancreatic cancer, and lung cancer. At present, low-dose CT scans may be of benefit for people who have a heavy smoking history (more than thirty pack years) and this is a weak recommendation in the US and Canada. Chest X-rays are not recommended as a screening test.

Unfortunately, we just do not have screening tests available for all conditions and, even with appropriate screening, we will still hear of unfortunate cases. No test is 100 percent without risk or can 100 percent guarantee the absence of cancer or a worrisome condition. Once again, uncertainty is something we all have to learn to accept in medicine and health. We can only do what we can and we have to try to be comfortable with that.

Summary

Trying to pick up a disease process before it causes symptoms and while treatment is viable is a worthwhile goal. Unfortunately, not many diseases fit the criteria for an effective screening program; even when they do, there are still risks and limitations that are important to be aware of. Thankfully, we have excellent organizations that evaluate evidence and provide recommendations for appropriate screening to consider.

The first priority is to focus on the actions that can help prevent and reduce the risk of developing these conditions. While it is no guarantee, following the lifestyle and behavior recommendations outlined in this book is the best way to reduce your risk.

The second priority is to consider the pros and cons of the available and recommended screening tests. In consultation with your physician, you can then decide what you feel comfortable with. Again, there are no guarantees, and uncertainty is the norm; all you can do is live the best life you can, get screening done when appropriate, and place your trust in that.

10

Supplement?

*"Be the kind of person who takes
supplements—then skip the supplements."*
Michael Pollan

WHEN PEOPLE ENVISION a "healthy" person, they usually picture someone who does much of what has been outlined here—and more. For some reason, the hard work of eating well, exercising, ensuring adequate sleep, and focusing on being happier—along with being a nonsmoker, getting vaccinated, and keeping up-to-date on appropriate screening tests—doesn't seem like it's enough.

Instead, there is this expectation that being *healthier* isn't sufficient; the goal is to be the *healthiest*. It's a contest to see who is eating the "cleanest," whose workout routine is the best, what vitamin cocktail is the most innovative, which "detox" is most effective, and how many other "maintenance" therapies can be done. Some people may have the time, energy, and money to pursue these things, but for those who do not, the impression that these additional measures are necessary can be frustrating, dejecting, and demoralizing.

Thankfully, the reality is that these additional products and actions are not required, often are of no benefit at all, and may actually cause some harm. Again, I think we need to realign our image of health from that of a celebrity or athlete who has unlimited resources and time to pursue the goal of looking good on a movie screen or gaining a slight advantage on the football field (and who likely has a personal trainer and chef), with that of a healthy eighty-year-old who is enjoying life and all of its pleasures in moderation. And while that celebrity or athlete may have extra motivation to try anything to look younger longer and be able to play better, all of that effort likely yields minimal benefit, if any, beyond the fundamentals we have already focused on (as well as good genetics and some luck).

As a verb, *supplement* means to add an extra amount to something; as a noun, it is something that adds or enhances something else. I like to think of it as something that is "in addition to"—so in regards to health, a supplemental therapy or vitamin should be considered *in addition to* an already healthy lifestyle.

If you have addressed all of the core elements of being healthy, as reviewed in chapters one to nine, then it could be reasonable to supplement. But if you are looking to use these items to substitute for healthy behaviors, like eating more fruits and vegetables or exercising, then your energy is being misplaced.

When talking about supplements, I am including various therapies that are used as general health measures rather than as treatments. This includes things like routine acupuncture, chiropractic adjustments, routine massage therapy, cleanses, detoxifications, Reiki, and other therapies that are marketed as part of regular health maintenance. I am not denying that there may be value in taking some time periodically to focus on you, or that these modalities may feel nice; I am saying that they are not *required* to be healthy and should be considered as "supplements," just as a vitamin would be.

So, assuming that you have already focused on the fundamentals of health and are considering adding supplements to your regimen, how do you decide what to do or take when there is so much offered and promoted as important to living well?

Start with a clear process to consider these additional therapies to help decide if the treatment makes sense for you or not. That process involves four basic questions:

1. What are the benefits?
2. What are the harms?
3. What are the costs?
4. How convenient is it?

What Are the Benefits?

The initial steps in assessing any supplement are similar to what we do when evaluating any health claim, as explained in the "Think" chapter.

Focus on the Claim Itself

When looking at a treatment, it is valuable to consider why you are even thinking of taking it. What benefit are you hoping to gain from it, and how will you know if it works? We can easily break down what we hope to get from any treatment, medication, or therapy to three basic factors:

- It helps us live longer.
- It helps us avoid major illness.
- It helps us feel better.

Marketing gives the impression that supplements can do all three; we need to be more specific. What is the actual claim being made? "It's good for you" isn't enough. Is it meant to prevent a type of cancer, help you feel less pain, or have more energy? Then focus on the evidence for that specific claim.

Determine Pre-test Probability

What is the likelihood that the proposed therapy is of any benefit given what we already know about health and science?

Check for Biases

Are you being swayed by your own biases and looking for information that confirms what you already believe? Does the person, group, or company making the claim have a conflict of interest or their own bias? Or is the evidence from a reliable, objective source?

Assess the Basis of the Claim

Is there replicable, high-quality evidence from double-blind, placebo-controlled, randomized clinical trials in support of the claim? Or is it based on anecdotes, celebrity endorsement, an appeal to nature, an appeal to ancient wisdom, or other weak logical arguments?

When looked at in this manner, there isn't much support for the promoted benefits of vitamins and many preventive maintenance therapies. Despite what we are continually told and sold, there has been lots of high-quality research done on a variety of vitamins and therapies that has consistently shown a lack of benefit and, at times, potential harm from these supplements. Whether it's vitamin C for colds, saw palmetto to protect the prostate, St.-John's-wort for depression, vitamin E for cancer prevention, or any of a multitude of claims regarding vitamins for various conditions—when these claims were studied, no evidence of benefit was found. Similarly, with other treatment modalities like chiropractic spine manipulations, acupuncture, and Reiki, there has been no difference shown between actual therapy and so-called sham therapy (doing similar motions without doing the actual treatment).

It needs to be noted that with most supplements there is *evidence demonstrating that there is no benefit*—research has shown them to be ineffective over placebo. It is not the same thing as saying there is *no evidence for benefit*—that no research has been done, so we don't know if it works or not. While there are certainly some things that have not been tested, research has been done for the vast majority of supplemental therapies, and the evidence is there to state that they are not necessary or beneficial.

Does this mean that we don't need vitamins? Certainly not. Vitamins and minerals are defined as groups of compounds that are required for growth and nutrition that we need to ingest since we are not able to make them ourselves. Vitamins are made by plants and animals, whereas minerals are inorganic and are absorbed or eaten by the foods we in turn eat. The question isn't whether we need them or not, but rather how much do we need and do we get any benefit from taking more? Study after study has shown that we do not need any more than is recommended by dietitians and that we can easily get them through our regular diet.

If you are deficient in something or at risk of being deficient, there may be value in taking supplements, although it would be best to focus on tackling the deficiency through your diet. The most common supplements in North America in specific situations are as follows:

- calcium and vitamin D in post-menopausal women and those at risk of fractures to help with bone strength

- adequate iron intake for those who are low in iron

- adequate vitamin B12 intake for those at risk (vegans, those over age fifty)

- vitamin D supplementation for infants who are breastfed

- folic acid intake (400 mcg/day) for women of childbearing age who are considering becoming pregnant to minimize risk of birth defects

- vitamin K for newborns to reduce risk of severe bleeding

Beyond those vitamins in those situations, research has not shown any real benefit from supplemental doses. Even with vitamin D and probiotics—in people who are not known to be deficient and have no symptoms—for which there have been numerous studies and some promising research, there still isn't anything conclusive enough to make a strong recommendation. A daily multivitamin generally contains the approximately recommended daily intakes of the various vitamins and minerals; people take them as a sort of backup policy to ensure they are getting what they need and this may be reasonable for some. In reality, however, most of us are already getting those minimums from our diet. If you do wish to improve your vitamin profile in any way, you would be better off focusing on what you get from food.

Dr. Michael Allan, a family doctor from Edmonton and co-host of the *Best Science Medicine* podcast, has a great line about the value of vitamins. He recommends that if you want to get the most benefit from them, bring them to a friend's house who lives about two miles away and leave them there. When it's time to take your vitamins, get up, walk over to your friend's place, swallow the pill, and walk back! And if you want even more benefit, pick a friend who lives farther away or consider mailing them to a country whose population has known vitamin deficiencies—Mongolia, for example.

To my mind, the benefit of supplements is just not there. I would always choose to improve my diet and increase my level of exercise, as I know that the return on my investment will be far greater. But that's my choice. If you still feel that pursuing such a treatment has value, then you need to consider the next question in our thought process—what about potential harms?

What Are the Harms?

Now that you have assessed what benefit you expect to get from a supplement and the rationale or evidence behind it, it is time to consider the potential harms. Any treatment, medication, or therapy that is expected to have some effect on the body also has the potential to create a side effect. And since most supplements have evidence of no benefit at all, the standards for safety must be incredibly high.

If a treatment has the potential to save your life, then you can tolerate a higher likelihood of side effects. Chemotherapy obviously has significant side effects, but if it has the chance to save your life, most of us are willing to accept that. In contrast, taking a substance that has been shown to have no effect or minimal benefit requires it to be, first and foremost, safe to take.

There are three major categories of potential harm to consider:

1. Harmful side effects of the product itself
2. Harmful effects of substances contaminating the product
3. Harmful interactions with other medications being taken

Each are concerning in their own way and worth keeping in mind.

1. Harmful Side Effects of the Product Itself

Some supplements and herbal products have known effects on the body. Again, just because something is natural does not mean that it is safe. And if you are taking something because you feel there is a benefit for your body, you must consider that it can also create some negative effects. The body does not care about the source of the substance—the body responds to the chemical, whether it comes from a plant or the lab. As Scott Gavura, a pharmacist and contributor to ScienceBasedMedicine.org, states, "Once we swallow a substance, be it a herb or a drug, our body can't distinguish the difference."

There are numerous examples of people being hurt by the medicinal properties of substances found in supplements. Aristolochia clematitis, which has been used for years for everything from headaches to weight loss, has been associated with significant kidney damage. Black cohosh and valerian root have both been known to affect the liver negatively. Echinacea has been linked with asthma, and saw palmetto might affect platelets and be associated with increased bleeding. There are numerous other examples of the potential harms of supplements; many of them have a chemical effect on the body.

A major concern with the supplement industry is that it is essentially unregulated. Due to significant campaigning by the massive companies that earn billions of dollars in this field, these products are not subject to the same standards as food and drugs. Even though millions of people ingest them daily, there is little regulation requiring safety testing or quality controls. While medicines are required to prove their effectiveness, demonstrate their safety, and then list any and all potential side effects, this reporting is not required of supplements—it doesn't mean the side effects don't exist.

Supplemental treatments also have the potential for risk. Manipulation of the neck has been reported to be a potential factor in dissection of the vertebral artery and cause of stroke. This risk is very small but, for a procedure with no proven benefit, any risk of such a catastrophic outcome needs to be considered. With other procedures that involve any kind of invasive action or the insertion of objects (enemas, vaginal inserts, even acupuncture needles), there can also be an associated risk that needs to be weighed against any potential benefit.

2. Harmful Effects of Substances Contaminating the Product

Due to the poor regulation of vitamins and herbal products, it is common for them to contain unexpected herbs or even drugs. Sometimes the beneficial effects of the product are due to the contaminants themselves. It is common knowledge that many of the alternative therapies offered at clinics in other countries contain steroids, which unsurprisingly can make people feel better and have powerful effects. Other common pharmaceutical contaminants in "natural" supplements include Viagra in aphrodisiacs, sedatives in sleep aids, and typical diabetes medication in herbal diabetic supplements.

In studies on supplements, common findings of contamination have been due to the insertion of unlabeled products, substitution of the main ingredient, mislabeling, and/or poor manufacturing standards. Some recent examples include:

- In 2005, a survey of Ayurvedic medicines found 20 percent were contaminated with heavy metals such as lead, mercury, and arsenic.

- In 2007, FDA regulators were allowed to supervise how supplements were being made in 450 manufacturing plants and found significant concerns in more than half of those inspected.

- In 2011, a study of 131 herbal teas found 33 percent were contaminated and only 58 percent could be authenticated.

- In 2013, a study of forty-four products found only 48 percent were authentic and 59 percent contained species of herbs not on the label. One-third contained a substituted ingredient—and none of the labeled one.

With this lack of oversight, it is hard to truly assess the potential harm of taking supplements. While it may well be a small risk, the uncertainty is unsettling. Given that the level of benefit is minimal, if present at all, it can be very hard to feel confident in the value of taking them.

3. Harmful Interactions with Other Medications Being Taken

Before taking supplements, consider that the herbs or substances in them may interact with other drugs you are also taking. Some potential interactions include:

- Vitamin E can increase the effect of warfarin, a blood thinner, and thus increase the risk of bleeding.

- Vitamin A taken in addition to some acne medications (tretinoins) can lead to vitamin A toxicity, which can cause nausea, vomiting, diarrhea, blurred vision, dizziness, and poor muscle coordination.

- Calcium can limit the absorption of some antibiotics if taken close in time to each other.

- St.-John's-wort has been demonstrated to interact with a number of medications including contraceptives, digoxin, warfarin, and benzodiazepines.

Given the potential for interaction of these substances with other prescribed medications, inform your pharmacist and physician of all that you are taking. Also, it is important that you do not stop your conventional medications without first discussing it in detail with your physician. Or you could contemplate whether this risk of interaction is worth whatever gains you are hoping to get from the supplement.

What Are the Costs?

After reviewing the potential benefits and harms of the supplemental therapy you are considering, the next issue to address is the cost. There are two main costs that need to be considered: financial costs and opportunity costs.

Financial Costs

As most of you are aware, the cost of supplements or other therapies is not trivial. In fact, the reason that we often associate people who do these additional things with good health is that *they are wealthy enough to afford them.* It is this increased financial status that is the driver for their health, not the supplements they are buying.

I often see patients in my practice spending *hundreds of dollars a month* on various supplements and treatments that are not making any significant difference to their well-being. Often they are simultaneously struggling with the cost of medications that have a proven benefit for their specific health condition. That money could also be better spent on any number of other things to directly improve their quality of life—better food, a gym membership, counseling, an emotionally satisfying hobby, or outings with friends.

Keeping the definition of supplement in mind, it may be reasonable to consider a supplement if you are acting on all the other fundamentals of good health, believe the potential benefits outweigh the harms, and can afford it. Perhaps then it may make sense for you to *add this* to your health regimen. But otherwise, I think that money would be far better used to go to a movie with a buddy.

Opportunity Costs

The other way that supplements may cost you is in lost opportunities. Sometimes people take supplements and vitamins in the belief that it's a substitute for healthy eating, physical activity, positive sleep hygiene, or conventional medicine. This is incorrect, not helpful to your overall health, and potentially harmful.

The most dangerous concern is that the use of supplements or alternative therapies may lead to the delay or avoidance of conventional therapy. Unfortunately, there are cases where people have died as a result of this choice. In 2012, a nineteen-month-old boy died of meningitis after being treated exclusively by naturopathic remedies; the parents were found guilty of failing to provide the necessities of life. While cases involving children are particularly upsetting, there are also numerous cases of adults trying alternative therapies prior to more evidence-based and effective traditional treatments. Depending on the illness involved, this choice can lead to unnecessary outcomes. In one small study of breast cancer patients who chose alternative methods rather than surgery—which can often be curative—five out of the six patients had progressed to stage IV before they followed up with the surgeons.

Thankfully, most people are not considering the use of supplements over conventional treatments for serious illnesses. The majority are just trying to be healthier and want to do what they can to achieve that. In that light, you need to consider the potential lost opportunity when you choose to spend

the time, money, and energy on these often-unproven therapies. In almost all cases, you would be better off focusing on
the fundamentals of health.

Ignore the noise and trust in what you know will make a difference. That is the best way to a healthier life—and it's likely
cheaper, easier, and more enjoyable as well.

How Convenient Is It?

The final factor to consider when assessing the value of additional supplements and treatments is the convenience of
them. This may seem silly in some ways; how hard is it to take
a vitamin in the morning? But in reality, it can be a nuisance to
take something daily. A few years ago, I tried to take vitamin
D daily—during the winter, since I live in Canada. As someone who doesn't usually take any pills, I found it very hard to
get into the habit. I eventually stopped trying due to the lack
of strong evidence for it and due to the tiny inconvenience. I
know many patients who struggle to take their prescribed medications, despite much better evidence, because of the same
inconvenience issue.

The regimen that some people are asked to follow, as recommended by naturopaths and alternative practitioners, can
be incredibly daunting and complicated. A prominent practitioner, Dr. Andrew Weil, who has fashioned himself as an
"integrative" health guru, graduated from Harvard Medical
School but dropped out of his residency and then established
an empire focused on alternative medicine. He promotes some
positive elements of healthy living but integrates a lot of questionable practices as well.

Let's look at his vitamin cocktail:

- In the morning, he takes a multivitamin, co-enzyme Q10, a mixed-mushroom supplement, magnesium, four fish oil capsules, acetyl-L-carnitine, and alpha-linoleic acid.

- In the evening, he takes another multivitamin, co-enzyme Q10, two vitamin D tablets, two baby aspirin, a mixed-mushroom supplement, magnesium, four fish oil capsules, acetyl-L-carnitine, and alpha-linoleic acid.

Weil also advises eating well, but I would have a hard time eating with all those supplements in me. And, as is typical, Dr. Weil recommends his own brand of these vitamins. The supplements recommended are often sold by the one giving the advice.

Beyond swallowing a lot of pills, many other maintenance and preventive health therapies involve much more inconvenience. Colonic irrigation, or cleaning out your bowels with warm water (or other products), is something I would consider to be fairly inconvenient and couldn't imagine doing it without a compelling reason.

"Cleanses" or "detoxes" often involve a very restrictive diet for a day, week, or longer together with a specific regimen of supplements. Any short-term drastic change is not going to have any significant beneficial effect on your health—you are far better to invest your energy in smaller, more effective changes that you can incorporate into your daily life. It is also important to note that the best detoxification is done by your functioning liver and kidneys; they will work hard to offset anything you try to do to alter the inner environment of your body.

Even maintenance therapies with acupuncturists, chiropractors, or other practitioners can be quite intrusive. It takes time to make an appointment, drive, park, and attend the session. That visit can take you away from work, family, friends, play, exercise, and other more worthwhile activities. Again, it is mainly those with the financial means and the time who can afford these types of therapies; time, money, and making wellness a priority are often the more relevant factors to health than the treatments themselves.

After you use this four-step process of assessing potential benefits, potential harms, the cost, and the level of (in)convenience, you may still choose to use particular supplemental products and treatments. My hope is that this process will make the decision easier and more conscious, given my experience that many people use them with very unclear hopes, goals, and rationale.

Why Are We Attracted to "Alternative" Therapies?

But why do we gravitate toward these kinds of therapies? What is it about them, or perhaps about conventional medicine, that makes them so appealing? The reasoning relates back to concepts discussed in the "Think" chapter as well as to some specific aspects of the supplement and complementary therapy world.

Natural & Ancient vs. Modern & Medical

Seeking alternative therapies with the idea that they are better because they are natural or derived from ancient practices—and therefore must be good—is an error in thinking that should be addressed. Again, it is reasonable to think about and consider alternatives, but I would advise you to use the structured process discussed in this chapter to consciously consider the pros and cons. If that process provides you with enough confidence to take it, then by all means do so. You are then taking something with your eyes wide open; doing so solely due to the natural or ancient fallacy can lead you down some unnecessary paths.

Holistic vs. Pill Pushers

When we hear about alternative health providers, a common term used is *holistic*, which is defined as the treatment of the whole person taking into account mental and social factors, rather than just the physical symptoms of a disease. I don't think you would find any medical doctor or practitioner who disagrees with this view of whole health. When it is used by other health providers, it often describes practitioners who are willing to use homeopathic medicine, acupuncture, herbal supplements, and other therapies not proven by science. Again, there is only one type of medicine—that which has been proven to work; otherwise it is not effective and not recommended.

Another element of this argument is that naturopaths and other practitioners focus more on lifestyle modification than drugs in addressing health concerns. Certainly, many physicians could do a better job of emphasizing diet and exercise as a means of healthy living. Again, no physician would discount the value of improving diet and activity in addressing all aspects of health; in fact, it is consistently the first-line treatment for any number of health conditions. This is not alternative medicine—a healthy diet and increased exercise is mainstream medicine and always has been.

But even if there is room for doctors to improve in the area of lifestyle advice, that is no reason to seek alternative therapies. The medical system can and should focus on doing a better job around that aspect of care, and patients seeking more support than their physician provides can look to registered dietitians and/or personal trainers in that regard.

Passive vs. Active

You may have noticed that much of what has been discussed in this book involves active participation on your part—exercising more, eating better, developing good sleep habits, quitting smoking, and being more invested in your own happiness. This is contrary to what is often seen in the alternative health market and even in conventional medicine. You need the help of external sources to achieve wellness, be that a practitioner laying their hands on you; taking a particular cocktail of vitamins, supplements, or prescriptions; or using a particular device.

I understand the appeal of that. When I suffered a back injury, all I wanted was someone to "do something to me" to make me feel better. But what I needed to do was to actively stretch and exercise to help my body recover. As much as we all say we want to avoid pills, at some point we will have that urge to take something to feel better. While there is certainly a role for medication in the treatment of numerous conditions, there is always a role for lifestyle interventions as well. And when you are looking at preventive measures when you are not sick, then doing something active will always be more effective than passive treatment.

It may be human nature to want to take a sleeping pill or a vitamin rather than work on sleep hygiene or improve our diet, but it is often better for our health to do the harder thing. The goal is to focus on what matters, and, as I've outlined in this book, these factors are important and worth the effort.

Certainty vs. Uncertainty

Another feature common to many alternative therapies and practices is that they convey a level of certainty that is not necessarily accurate. It would be nice to know exactly why one has back pain or developed cancer or had a heart attack, but it's often not possible. People may do everything "right" and still develop serious health problems. "Why?" is typically a very hard question to answer.

Certainty—in both diagnosis and treatment—is communicated by the alternative health community, while the traditional medical system tends to talk in terms of probability, risk reduction, and numbers needed to treat. This uncertainty is much harder to communicate, is much less satisfying, and harder to comprehend. But it is more accurate. When you are trying any treatments or interventions, you are reducing the risk; there are no guarantees.

I understand how certainty suggests confidence and reliability. As medical practitioners, we often choose our words in such a way to foster belief in our treatments and perhaps boost the placebo response of an already proven treatment. The problem arises when there is little evidence to back up that declaration of certainty.

I also worry about patients feeling that they are to blame: "I got cancer because I didn't take the right vitamins, eat the right foods, or do the right thing." That isn't fair or correct. It isn't right to put that blame on patients. Health, and life in general, is full of uncertainty. Focus on what you *can* do to be well and reduce your risk of getting a serious illness. Beyond that, you have to let go of your anxieties and do something really difficult— trust that it will be okay. Thankfully, in most cases, it will be.

Hope vs. Reality

Similar to the issue with certainty, the sometimes-cold reality of facts and figures presented by the medical profession can be a stark contrast to the hope provided by alternative practitioners, particularly for people dealing with a significant illness. There are numerous conditions for which effective cures or treatments are lacking—many cancers, dementia, multiple sclerosis, Lou Gehrig's disease, and fibromyalgia, for example—and thus there is a market for alternative treatments. Hope definitely sells.

In contrast, we physicians have to discuss the harsh truths about these conditions. While we never want to remove hope from the equation, we have a responsibility to be truthful. There may not be a cure, but we can help alleviate symptoms. We won't drain bank accounts with ineffective therapies but will rather focus on maintaining quality of life while managing terminal conditions. We can offer treatments that may not cure a chronic condition but may help control symptoms and improve function. None of this is sexy, but it is real.

I can only imagine the horror of having a sick child and wanting to do anything you can to help them. But I can never imagine offering ineffective treatments to vulnerable patients looking for a cure that doesn't exist. If any treatment does show promise, then it needs to be studied accurately and then offered to *all people* who would benefit. Keeping these "miracle" cures only available to those who can afford them is questionable behavior to me in a lot of ways.

Celebrity & Charisma vs. Facts & Numbers

Keeping with the theme that those of us in the medical profession are not sexy, the proponents of many alternative therapies are often celebrities or practitioners with charismatic personalities. Look at Dr. Mehmet Oz, Jenny McCarthy, Tom Brady, Gwyneth Paltrow, Dr. Deepak Chopra, and any number of other celebrities like the Kardashians and Katy Perry who promote lifestyle and health advice. While some may be charismatic physicians with their own particular view on health, most are simply famous and promote their ideas based on their own experience or for handsome fees.

These additional things they do and promote are window dressings on an already healthy lifestyle. Keep in mind that the images you see of them are typically modified and that they don't often mention other treatments they may receive, such as Botox injections, surgical facelifts, and nonsurgical facial rejuvenation therapies.

What About Psychotherapy?

Psychotherapy, counseling, psychodynamic therapy, cognitive behavioral therapy, acceptance and commitment therapy, and numerous other forms of talk therapy are available to help people with their moods, emotions, stress management strategies, and life in general. This is a challenging area to get good evidence due to the variable and individualized nature of the therapeutic relationship. Some modalities are easier to study because of a more structured nature, but it may not mean that they are better than other more psychodynamic approaches.

One of the most important influences on the effectiveness of these techniques may well be the relationship and trust you have with your practitioner. And while there may be a lot of similar benefit to talking with a trusted friend, there likely is value in having a nonjudgmental third party who has some specialized training in emotional guidance and management.

Be wary of the potential for pseudoscience in this field, but for many patients, the time spent on focusing on their mental health is invaluable.

Summary

While supplementing may seem like a necessary step to a healthy life, the evidence suggests otherwise. This should be a relief to many of you, as it can free up time and money for other activities far more beneficial for your body and mind.

When considering taking any additional supplement to increase your overall wellness, it is prudent to go through a structured process to determine whether it makes sense for you.

1. What are the benefits?
2. What are the harms?
3. What are the costs?
4. How convenient is it?

If that process satisfies you, then proceed. At present, there does not seem to be enough evidence to promote any vitamin supplement on a population level other than those specific scenarios discussed earlier. Even a daily multivitamin is not likely of value (although likely of little harm). Focus on the staples of eating well, exercising, sleeping enough, enjoying life, being a nonsmoker, being vaccinated, and screening appropriately— and let the rest go. If you follow those basic tenets of health, the benefit of any supplement is tiny and likely not worth the effort.

Conclusion

SINCE YOU'VE TAKEN the time to read this book, I imagine that you have an interest in improving your health and are looking for ways to do that. You've made the all-important first decision: to find ways to live better.

Hopefully, *Healthier You* has helped you on that quest by breaking down health to its fundamental components so you can focus your energy on those things that truly matter and then relax about all the rest. The wellness industry can make it seem incredibly complicated and expensive to live your best life when, in reality, the concepts are fairly simple and inexpensive.

Think. Change. Eat. Move. Sleep. Enjoy. Quit. Vaccinate. Screen. Supplement?

These are what I believe to be the most basic and essential aspects of health, and it's in these areas that we all could likely improve our efforts to be healthy. There are a number of evidence-based strategies to use within each category to increase your well-being. Very few people could honestly say that they can make no further progress in any of these facets of life.

There is no reason to resort to other time-consuming, expensive, and unproven therapies when there are so many practical things to do in order to live your best life. Focusing your efforts on even one category can make a huge difference to your health and improve your sense of well-being.

Think. By taking into account the numerous logical fallacies and cognitive biases we all have, you can cut through all of the confusing and nonsensical health claims out there and allow yourself to focus on the things that make the biggest difference to your health. It's like having a superpower that many people choose to ignore.

Change. Harness the science and psychology of change management to find your personal motivation to be healthier, direct your energy with SMART goals, and adjust your surroundings and mindset to optimize your chances of success. Rather than spinning your wheels with a vague idea of living better, you can start making practical strides to achieve that goal.

Eat. Use the basic principles of healthy eating as the basis for your dietary lifestyle. Focus on specific and proven eating behaviors in order to achieve your dietary and weight goals. Stick to the outside aisles of the grocery store. Try to cook more and eat out less. Consume mostly plants, being aware of how many calories you are eating. Minimize processed foods, liquid calories, and prepared items. But always remember that a healthy diet is only effective if it is sustainable, so you need to strive for the healthiest diet that you can mindfully enjoy—and whatever weight that leads to is just fine.

Move. Take advantage of one of the best health interventions out there by getting as much physical activity as you can. Get moving by standing more, using the stairs, parking farther away, and any other way you can make your regular day *harder*. Use SMART/FITT goals to include as much regular *enjoyable* exercise into your week as possible—knowing that any amount counts and more is probably better.

Sleep. Don't underestimate the value of getting sufficient and quality sleep. Use the science of good sleep hygiene to make sleep the priority it deserves to be. Go to bed and get up at the same times every day. Do not confuse your body; the bedroom is for sleep and "recreation," not TV, working, heavy discussions, texting, or social media. Aim for at least seven hours a night, and your body and health will thank you.

Enjoy. Being healthy isn't that important if you're not happy. Knowing that 40 percent of your happiness is determined by your own choices and behaviors, you can now make concrete steps to improve your levels of happiness: find your purpose, focus on gratitude, be kind to others, be a lifelong learner, savor the joys in life, connect with people, and develop your self-acceptance as well as your self-compassion. Rather than trying to be less miserable, you can focus on the positive outlook of becoming happier.

Quit. To no one's surprise, smoking is one of the worst things you can do for your health, so freeing yourself from your tobacco addiction must then be one of the best things you can do for your body. Smoking is body pollution and there is no reason to do it beyond relieving a sense of withdrawal. If you don't smoke, never start; if you do, make the effort to quit and do not give up on giving it up.

Vaccinate. After decades of vaccinations and millions upon millions of doses worldwide, the science is clear: *vaccines are safe and they work*. While there are those who are convinced of their harms, keep in mind the common errors in thinking involved in those arguments against vaccination. There is no debate on this among scientists, physicians, public health organizations, or governments worldwide. Protect yourself, your family, and your community by keeping up-to-date on your immunizations.

Screen. If you cannot prevent illness outright, then detecting disease before you have any symptoms and when it is minor or more treatable is the next best thing. While that seems reasonable, there are only a few conditions where this is a practical strategy. Given that, your best chance of avoiding disease overall is to still focus on the specific healthy behaviors outlined above. However, specific screening may be beneficial so do talk to your doctor about recommended screening for your age group and the pros and potential cons of testing.

Supplement? Using supplemental products or therapies in your quest to live a healthier life may seem reasonable to some of you. If so, by definition these should be *in addition to* the other priorities outlined above. Given the variety of promoted supplements and therapies, it is prudent to use a structured process to weigh their usefulness. Consider the specific benefit you are hoping to get, the quality of the evidence, the potential for harm, the cost of the treatment, and the convenience in your evaluation.

While these ten fundamental features of a healthy life can seem somewhat straightforward at times, they are not always easy. That's okay. These challenges shouldn't be intimidating though—see them as motivating since they are things that you can undertake right away to start improving your health today.

And even if it is sometimes hard, it is much more effective and efficient than wasting your time, energy, and money on things that have very little, if any, benefit toward your health. Also remember that your goal is the *healthiest life you can enjoy*. Always. Keep looking for ways to improve your health by adding to the joy, energy, love, and laughter you experience. Suffering and tolerance should not be central components in your pursuit of wellness.

Life is a gift and you owe it to yourself to enjoy it now and for as long as you can. Trust that these basic changes can and will have a profound impact on your health.

Here's to your health and happiness.

Selected Resources

Think
Foundation for Critical Thinking: criticalthinking.org
Critical Thinking Tutorial: philosophy.hku.hk/think

Change
Heath Brothers' Switch Resources: heathbrothers.com/
resources

Eat
The Diet Fix calculator: thedietfix.com/calculator.aspx
Calorie calculator on Calculator.net: calculator.net/calorie-
calculator.html
CalorieKing: calorieking.com
Spark People: sparkpeople.com
My Fitness Pal: myfitnesspal.com
My Net Diary: mynetdiary.com
Canadian Obesity Network: obesitynetwork.ca

Move

National Health Service's Couch to 5K: nhs.uk/LiveWellc25k/
Pages/couch-to-5k.aspx

Steve Speirs's One Hundred Pushups: hundredpushups.com/

The Twenty Pullups Challenge: twentypullups.com/

Zen Muscle Building/Toning Challenge: available in app
stores

StrongLifts 5×5 Workout Program for Beginners: stronglifts.
com/5x5/

Sleep

Sleep Cycle Alarm Clock: sleepcycle.com

Sleep Better: available in app stores

Sleeptracker: available in app stores

National Sleep Foundation's Official Sleep Diary:
sleepfoundation.org/content/nsf-official-sleep-diary

Enjoy

Action for Happiness: actionforhappiness.org

FranklinCovey Mission Statement Builder: msb.
franklincovey.com

Quit

Free tools and support: smokefree.gov and smokershelpline.ca

Vaccinate

Vaccination schedule (WHO): who.int/immunization/policy/
Immunization_routine_table1.pdf?ua=1

Vaccination schedule (Canada): canada.ca/en/public-health/
services/provincial-territorial-immunization-information/
provincial-territorial-routine-vaccination-programs-
infants-children.html

Screen

Screening recommendations (Canada): canadiantaskforce.
ca/guidelines/published-guidelines
Screening recommendations (USA):
uspreventiveservicestaskforce.org/Page/Name/
uspstf-a-and-b-recommendations
Choosing Wisely: choosingwisely.org

Supplement?

Science-Based Medicine: www.sciencebasedmedicine.org
National Center for Complementary and Integrative
Medicine: nccih.nih.gov/health/supplements

References

Chapter 1: Think

Bausell, R. Barker. *Snake Oil Science: The Truth about Complementary and Alternative Medicine.* New York: Oxford University Press, 2009.

Ellenberg, Jordan. *How Not to Be Wrong: The Power of Mathematical Thinking.* New York: Penguin Books, 2015.

Offit, Paul A. *Do You Believe in Magic?: Vitamins, Supplements, and All Things Natural: A Look Behind the Curtain.* New York: HarperCollins, 2014.

Sagan, Carl. *The Demon-Haunted World: Science as a Candle in the Dark.* New York: Random House Publishing Group, 1996.

Singh, Simon, and Edzard Ernst. *Trick or Treatment: Alternative Medicine on Trial.* London: Transworld, 2009.

Chapter 2: Change

Baumeister, Roy F., Ellen Bratslavsky, Mark Muraven, and Dianne M. Tice. "Ego Depletion: Is the Active Self a Limited Resource?" *Journal of Personality and Social Psychology* 74, no. 5 (1998): 1252–1265. doi:10.1037/0022-3514.74.5.1252.

Baumeister, Roy F., and John Tierney. *Willpower: Rediscovering the Greatest Human Strength.* New York: Penguin Books, 2012.

Dreifus, Claudia. "Zoologist Gives a Voice to Big Cats in the Wilderness." *New York Times,* December 18, 2007, nytimes.com/2007/12/18/science/18conv.html.

Duhigg, Charles. *The Power of Habit: Why We Do What We Do in Life and Business.* New York: Random House, 2012.

Dweck, Carol S. *Mindset: The New Psychology of Success*. New York: Ballantine Books, 2016.

Engber, Daniel. "A Whole Field of Psychology Research May Be Bunk. Scientists Should Be Terrified." *Slate*, March 6, 2016, slate.com/articles/ health_and_science/cover_story/2016/03/ego_depletion_an_influential_ theory_in_psychology_may_have_just_been_debunked.html.

Frankl, Viktor E. *Man's Search for Ultimate Meaning*. London: Random House, 2011.

Haidt, Jonathan. *The Happiness Hypothesis: Putting Ancient Wisdom to the Test of Modern Science*. London: Arrow Books, 2006.

Heath, Chip, and Dan Heath. *Switch: How to Change Things When Change Is Hard*. New York: Random House, 2013.

Kotter, John Paul, and Dan S. Cohen. *The Heart of Change: Real-Life Stories of How People Change Their Organizations*. Boston, MA: Harvard Business Review Press, 2012.

Levav, Jonathan, Mark Heitmann, Andreas Herrmann, and Sheena S. Iyengar. "Order in Product Customization Decisions: Evidence from Field Experiments." *Journal of Political Economy* 118, no. 2 (2010): 274–299. doi:10.1086/652463.

O'Leary, John. *On Fire: The 7 Choices to Ignite a Radically Inspired Life*. New York: North Star Way, 2016.

Pink, Daniel H. *Drive: The Surprising Truth about What Motivates Us*. New York: Riverhead Books, 2012.

Rabinowitz, Alan. "Dr. Alan Rabinowitz Part 2." SchneiderSpeech, July 21, 2010. Video, 9:42. youtube.com/watch?v=Ng2IfiVRex4.

Rabinowitz, Alan. "Dr. Alan Rabinowitz Story Part 1." SchneiderSpeech, July 21, 2010. Video, 6:10. youtube.com/watch?v=s4xruGov4jM.

Thaler, Richard H., and Cass R. Sunstein. *Nudge: Improving Decisions about Health, Wealth, and Happiness*. New York: Penguin Books, 2009.

Chapter 3: Eat

Brown Medical School and the Miriam Hospital Weight Control & Diabetes Research Center. "NWCR Facts." National Weight Control Registry. Accessed March 26, 2018. nwcr.ws/Research/default.htm.

Canadian Centre on Substance Abuse and Addiction. "Canada's Low-Risk Alcohol Drinking Guidelines." 2017. ccsa.ca/Resource%20Library/2012-Canada-Low-Risk-Alcohol-Drinking-Guidelines-Brochure-en.pdf.

Centers for Disease Control and Prevention. "Fact Sheets—Moderate Drinking." Alcohol and Public Health. Updated July 25, 2017. cdc.gov/ alcohol/fact-sheets/moderate-drinking.htm.

Centers for Disease Control and Prevention. "NCCDPHP: Community Health." National Center for Chronic Disease Prevention and Health Promotion. Updated March 13, 2017. cdc.gov/nccdphp/dch/multimedia/infographics/ newabnormal.htm.

Church, Timothy S., Diana M. Thomas, Catrine Tudor-Locke, Peter T. Katzmarzyk, Conrad P. Earnest, Ruben Q. Rodarte, Corby K. Martin, Steven N. Blair, and Claude Bouchard. "Trends over 5 Decades in U.S. Occupation-Related Physical Activity and Their Associations with Obesity." *PLoS ONE* 6, no. 5 (2011): e19657. doi.org/10.1371/journal.pone.0019657.

Fell, James, and Margaret Yúfera-Leitch. *Lose It Right: A Brutally Honest, 3-Stage Program to Help You Get Fit and Lose Weight Without Losing Your Mind*. Toronto: Random House Canada, 2014.

Freedhoff, Yoni, and Arya M. Sharma. *Best Weight: A Practical Guide to Office-Based Obesity Management*. Edmonton: The Canadian Obesity Network, 2010.

Freedhoff, Yoni. *The Diet Fix: Why Diets Fail and How to Make Yours Work*. Toronto: Random House Canada, 2015.

Harvard T.H. Chan School of Public Health. "Healthy Eating Plate & Healthy Eating Pyramid." The Nutrition Source. Accessed March 8, 2018. hsph. harvard.edu/nutritionsource/healthy-eating-plate/.

Hollis, Jack F., Christina M. Gullion, Victor J. Stevens, Phillip J. Brantley, Lawrence J. Appel, Jamy D. Ard, Catherine M. Champagne, *et al.* "Weight Loss During the Intensive Intervention Phase of the Weight-Loss Maintenance Trial." *American Journal of Preventive Medicine* 35, no. 2 (2008): 118-126. doi:10.1016/j.amepre.2008.04.013.

Kennedy, Ann Blair, Carl J. Lavie, and Steven N. Blair. "Fitness or Fatness." *Jama* 319, no. 3 (2018): 231. doi:10.1001/jama.2017.21649.

Magnuson, Bernadene, George Burdock, John Doull, R.M. Kroes, Gary Marsh, M.W. Pariza, Peter Spencer, W.J. Waddell, R. Walker, and Gary Williams. "Aspartame: A Safety Evaluation Based on Current Use Levels, Regulations, and Toxicological and Epidemiological Studies." *Critical Reviews in Toxicology* 37, no. 8 (2007): 629-727. doi:10.1080/10408440701516184.

National Institute on Alcohol Abuse and Alcoholism. "Alcohol Calorie Calculator." Accessed February 25, 2018. rethinkingdrinking.niaaa.nih.gov/ tools/Calculators/calorie-calculator.aspx.

Ogden, Cynthia L., Margaret D. Carroll, Brian K. Kit, and Katherine M. Flegal. "Prevalence of Obesity among Adults: United States, 2011-2012." U.S. Department of Health and Human Services, Centers for Disease Control and Prevention, National Center for Health Statistics, 2013.

Park, Madison. "Twinkie Diet Helps Nutrition Professor Lose 27 Pounds." CNN. November 8, 2010. cnn.com/2010/HEALTH/11/08/twinkie.diet. professor/index.html.

Pollan, Michael. *In Defense of Food: An Eater's Manifesto.* London: Penguin Books, 2009.

Rath, Tom. *Eat Move Sleep: How Small Choices Lead to Big Changes.* Arlington: Missionday, 2013.

Swinburn, Boyd, Gary Sacks, and Eric Ravussin. "Increased Food Energy Supply Is More Than Sufficient to Explain the US Epidemic of Obesity." *The American Journal of Clinical Nutrition* 90, no. 6 (2009): 1453–1456. doi:10.3945/ajcn.2009.28595.

Westerterp, Klass R. "Physical Activity and Physical Activity Induced Energy Expenditure in Humans: Measurement, Determinants, and Effects." *Frontiers in Physiology* 4 (April 2013). doi:10.3389/fphys.2013.00090.

Westerterp, Klass R., and J.R. Speakman. "Physical Activity Energy Expenditure Has Not Declined Since the 1980s and Matches Energy Expenditures of Wild Mammals." *International Journal of Obesity* 32, no. 8 (2008): 1256–1263. doi:10.1038/ijo.2008.74.

Chapter 4: Move

Asmundson, Gordon J.G., Mathew G. Fetzner, Lindsey B. Deboer, Mark B. Powers, Michael W. Otto, and Jasper A.J. Smits. "Let's Get Physical: A Contemporary Review of the Anxiolytic Effects of Exercise for Anxiety and Its Disorders." *Depression and Anxiety* 30, no. 4 (2013): 362–373. doi:10.1002/da.22043.

Beckerman, James. *Heart to Start: The Eight Week Exercise Prescription to Live Longer, Beat Heart Disease, and Run Your Best Race.* Portland: Providence Heart and Vascular Institute, 2015.

Biswas, Aviroop, Paul I. Oh, Guy E. Faulkner, Ravi R. Bajaj, Michael A. Silver, Marc S. Mitchell, and David A. Alter. "Sedentary Time and Its Association with Risk for Disease Incidence, Mortality, and Hospitalization in Adults." *Annals of Internal Medicine* 162, no. 2 (2015): 123. doi:10.7326/m14-1651.

Canadian Society for Exercise Physiology. "Guidelines." CSEP. 2011. Accessed February 25, 2018. csepguidelines.ca.

Cox, Carla E. "Role of Physical Activity for Weight Loss and Weight Maintenance." *Diabetes Spectrum* 30, no. 3 (2017): 157–160. doi:10.2337/ds17-0013.

Diaz, Keith M., Virginia J. Howard, Brent Hutto, Natalie Colabianchi, John E. Vena, Monika M. Safford, Steven N. Blair, and Steven P. Hooker. "Patterns of Sedentary Behavior and Mortality in U.S. Middle-Aged and Older Adults."

Annals of Internal Medicine 167, no. 7 (December 2017): 465. doi:10.7326/m17-0212.

Evans Health Lab. MakeYourDayHarder.com. Accessed February 25, 2018.

Evans, Mike. "23 and 1/2 Hours: What Is the Single Best Thing We Can Do for Our Health?" DocMikeEvans, December 2, 2011. Video, 9:18. youtube.com/watch?v=aUaInS6HIGo.

Evans, Mike. "Movember and Dr. Mike: Diagnosing and Treating Sitting Disease." DocMikeEvans, October 1, 2013. Video, 5:02. youtube.com/watch?v=QQRIaFqUPeQ.

Geneen, Louise J., R. Andrew Moore, Clare Clarke, Denis Martin, Lesley A. Colvin, and Blair H. Smith. "Physical Activity and Exercise for Chronic Pain in Adults: An Overview of Cochrane Reviews." *Cochrane Database of Systematic Reviews* 4 (2017). doi:10.1002/14651858.cd011279.pub3.

Haskell, William L., Steven N. Blair, and James O. Hill. "Physical Activity: Health Outcomes and Importance for Public Health Policy." *Preventive Medicine* 49, no. 4 (2009): 280–282. doi:10.1016/j.ypmed.2009.05.002.

Hayashi, Tomoshige, Kei Tsumura, Chika Suematsu, Kunio Okada, Satoru Fujii, and Ginji Endo. "Walking to Work and the Risk for Hypertension in Men: The Osaka Health Survey." *Annals of Internal Medicine* 131, no. 1 (1999): 21. doi:10.7326/0003-4819-131-1-199907060-00005.

Health Canada. "Health Status of Canadians 2016: Report of the Chief Public Health Officer What Is Influencing Our Health? Physical Activity." Canada.ca. Updated December 15, 2016. canada.ca/en/public-health/corporate/publications/chief-public-health-officer-reports-state-public-health-canada/2016-health-status-canadians/page-13-what-influencing-health-physical-activity.html.

Howard, Jacqueline. "Americans at More than 10 Hours a Day on Screens." CNN, July 29, 2016. cnn.com/2016/06/30/health/americans-screen-time-nielsen/index.html.

Hutchinson, Alex. *Which Comes First, Cardio or Weights?: Fitness Myths, Training Truths, and Other Surprising Discoveries from the Science of Exercise.* New York: HarperCollins, 2011.

Leitzmann, Michael F. "Physical Activity Recommendations and Decreased Risk of Mortality." *Archives of Internal Medicine* 167, no. 22 (2007): 2453. doi:10.1001/archinte.167.22.2453.

Loprinzi, Paul D., and Bradley J. Cardinal. "Association between Objectively-Measured Physical Activity and Sleep, NHANES 2005-2006." *Mental Health and Physical Activity* 4, no. 2 (2011): 65–69. doi:10.1016/j.mhpa.2011.08.001.

Penedo, Frank J., and Jason R. Dahn. "Exercise and Well-Being: A Review of Mental and Physical Health Benefits Associated with Physical Activity." *Current Opinion in Psychiatry* 18, no. 2 (2005): 189-193. doi:10.1097/00001504-200503000-00013.

Penninx, Brenda W.J.H., Stephen P. Messier, W. Jack Rejeski, Jeff D. Williamson, Mauro DiBari, Chiara Cavazzini, William B. Applegate, and Marco Pahor. "Physical Exercise and the Prevention of Disability in Activities of Daily Living in Older Persons with Osteoarthritis." *Archives of Internal Medicine* 161, no. 19 (2001): 2309-2316. doi:10.1001/archinte.161.19.2309.

Perše, Martina. "Physical Activity, Dietary Fat and Colorectal Cancer." In *Colorectal Cancer—From Prevention to Patient Care*. IntechOpen, February 17, 2012. doi:10.5772/27462.

"Physical Fitness." *New World Encyclopedia*. Updated February 12, 2015. newworldencyclopedia.org/entry/Physical_fitness.

Rath, Linda. "Osteoarthritis Prevention: What You Can Do." Arthriti Foundation. Accessed February 25, 2018. arthritis.org/about-arthritis/types/osteoarthritis/articles/oa-prevention.php.

Rippetoe, Mark, and Stephani Elizabeth Bradford. *Starting Strength: Basic Barbell Training*. Wichita Falls, TX: Aasgaard Company, 2017.

Warburton, Darren E.R., Crystal Whitney Nicol, and Shannon S.D. Bredin. "Health Benefits of Physical Activity: The Evidence." *Canadian Medical Association Journal* 174, no. 6 (March 2006): 801-809. doi:10.1503/cmaj.051351.

Warburton, Darren E.R., Veronica K. Jamnik, Shannon S.D. Bredin, and Norman Gledhill. "The Physical Activity Readiness Questionnaire (PAR-Q+) and Electronic Physical Activity Readiness Medical Examination (EPARmed-X+)." *Health & Fitness Journal of Canada* 4, no.2 (April 14, 2011): 3-23. new-hfjc.library.ubc.ca/index.php/html/article/download/103/66.

Yates, Thomas, Melanie Davies, and Kamlesh Khunti. "Prevention of Type 2 Diabetes: The Role of Physical Activity." *Prevention of Diabetes* (2013): 159-176. doi:10.1002/9781118661321.ch11.

Chapter 5: Sleep

Allan, G. Michael, and Jobin Varughese. "Trouble Sleeping: Spend Less Time in Bed?" Tools for Practice, Alberta College of Family Physicians, May 29 2017, acfp.ca/wp-content/uploads/tools-for-practice/1495207198_tfp188sleeprestrictionfv2.pdf.

Chaput, Jean-Philippe, Suzy L. Wong, and Isabelle Michaud. "Duration and Quality of Sleep Among Canadians Aged 18 to 79." Statistics Canada. September 20, 2017. statcan.gc.ca/pub/82-003-x/2017009/article/54857-eng.htm.

Glass, Jennifer, Krista L. Lanctôt, Nathan Herrmann, Beth A. Sproule, and Usoa E. Busto. "Sedative Hypnotics in Older People with Insomnia: Meta-Analysis of Risks and Benefits." *BMJ* 331, no. 7526 (2005): 1169. doi:10.1136/bmj.38623.768588.47.

Hauri, Peter, and Shirley Linde. *No More Sleepless Nights.* New York: Wiley, 1996.

Holbrook, Anne M., Reneé Crowther, Ann Lotter, Chiachen Cheng, and Derek King. "Meta-analysis of Benzodiazepine Use in the Treatment of Insomnia." *CMAJ: Canadian Medical Association Journal* 162, no. 2 (2000): 225-233.

Jacobs, Gregg D. *Say Good Night to Insomnia.* New York: Henry Holt, 2009.

Kaiser Permanente. "Sleep Restriction Therapy." thrive.kaiserpermanente. org/care-near-you/northern-california/sanjose/wp-content/uploads/ sites/7/2015/10/sleep-restriction-rev2_tcm28-557887.pdf.

Lee, Rebecca. "Consumer Reports: What Sleep Remedies Actually Work?" CBS News, January 11, 2016, cbsnews.com/news/ consumer-reports-investigation-sleeping-aids-remedies/.

Morin, Charles M., Richard R. Bootzin, Daniel J. Buysse, Jack D. Edinger, Colin A. Espie, and Kenneth L. Lichstein. "Psychological and Behavioral Treatment of Insomnia: Update of the Recent Evidence (1998-2004)." *Sleep* 29, no. 11 (November 1, 2006): 1398-1414. doi:10.1093/ sleep/29.11.1398.

National Institutes of Health. "Melatonin: In Depth." National Center for Complementary and Integrative Health. Updated September 24, 2017. nccih.nih.gov/health/melatonin.

National Sleep Foundation. "What Is Insomnia?" Sleep Foundation. Accessed February 26, 2018. sleepfoundation.org/insomnia/content/ what-is-insomnia.

Reframe Health Lab. "Sleeping Better." Accessed February 26, 2018. ReframeHealthLab.com/sleeping/.

Sleep Research Society. "Practice Parameters for the Psychological and Behavioral Treatment of Insomnia: An Update. An American Academy of Sleep Medicine Report." *Sleep* 29, no. 11 (November 1, 2006): 1415-1419. doi:10.1093/sleep/29.11.1415.

Working on the Moon. "Sleep." Updated October 13, 2010. workingonthemoon.com/WOTM-Sleep.html.

Chapter 6: Enjoy

Achor, Shawn. *The Happiness Advantage: The Seven Principles that Fuel Success and Performance at Work.* London: Virgin, 2011.

Action for Happiness. "10 Keys to Happier Living." Accessed March 26, 2018. actionforhappiness.org/10-keys.

Action for Happiness. "Let's Take Action for a Happier World." Accessed February 27, 2018. actionforhappiness.org.

Ben-Shahar, Tal. *Happier: Learn the Secrets to Daily Joy and Lasting Fulfillment.* New York: McGraw-Hill, 2007.

Berges, Ivonne-Marie, Gary Seale, and Glenn V. Ostir. "Positive Affect and Pain Ratings in Persons with Stroke." *Rehabilitation Psychology* 56, no. 1 (2011): 52-57. doi:10.1037/a0022683.

Cohen, Sheldon, William J. Doyle, Ronald B. Turner, Cuneyt M. Alper, and David P. Skoner. "Emotional Style and Susceptibility to the Common Cold." *Psychosomatic Medicine* 65, no. 4 (2003): 652-657. doi:10.1097/01. psy.0000077508.57784.da.

Csikszentmihalyi, Mihaly. *Flow: The Psychology of Optimal Experience.* New York: Harper Row, 2009.

Danner, Deborah D., David A. Snowdon, and Wallace V. Friesen. "Positive Emotions in Early Life and Longevity: Findings from the Nun Study." *Journal of Personality and Social Psychology* 80, no. 5 (2001): 804-813. doi:10.1037/0022-3514.80.5.804.

Davidson, Karina W., Elizabeth Mostofsky, and William Whang. "Don't Worry, Be Happy: Positive Affect and Reduced 10-Year Incident Coronary Heart Disease: The Canadian Nova Scotia Health Survey." *European Heart Journal* 31, no. 9 (2010): 1065-1070. doi:10.1093/eurheartj/ehp603.

Frankl, Viktor E. *Man's Search for Ultimate Meaning.* London: Random House, 2011.

FranklinCovey. "Personal Mission Statement Examples." Mission Statement Builder. Accessed March 8, 2018. msb.franklincovey.com/.

Headey, Bruce. "The Set Point Theory of Well-being Has Serious Flaws: On the Eve of a Scientific Revolution?" *Social Indicators Research* 97, no. 1 (2010): 7-21. doi:10.1007/s11205-009-9559-x.

Kahneman, Daniel. "Would You Be Happier If You Were Richer? A Focusing Illusion." *Science* 312, no. 5782 (2006): 1908-1910. doi:10.1126/science.1129688.

Kahneman, Daniel, and Angus Deaton. "High Income Improves Evaluation of Life but Not Emotional Well-being." *Proceedings of the National Academy of Sciences* 107, no. 38 (2010): 16489-16493.

Kroenke, Kurt, Robert L. Spitzer, and Janet B.W. Williams. "The PHQ-9: Validity of a Brief Depression Severity Measure." *Journal of General Internal Medicine* 16, no. 9 (September 2001):606-613. doi:10.1046/j.1525-1497.2001.016009606.x.

Lyubomirsky, Sonja, Kennon M. Sheldon, and David Schkade. "Pursuing Happiness: The Architecture of Sustainable Change." *Review of General Psychology* 9, no. 2 (2005):111-131. doi:10.1037/1089-2680.9.2.111.

Lyubomirsky, Sonja. *The How of Happiness: A New Approach to Getting the Life You Want*. New York: Penguin Books, 2008.

Seligman, Martin E.P. *Flourish: A Visionary New Understanding of Happiness and Well-being*. North Sydney, NSW: Random House Australia, 2012.

White, Daniel K., Julie J. Keysor, Tuhina Neogi, David T. Felson, Michael Lavalley, K. Doug Gross, Jingbo Niu, *et al.* "When It Hurts, a Positive Attitude May Help: Association of Positive Affect with Daily Walking in Knee Osteoarthritis. Results from a Multicenter Longitudinal Cohort Study." *Arthritis Care & Research* 64, no. 9 (2012):1312-1319. doi:10.1002/acr.21694.

Chapter 7: Quit

Allan, G. Michael, Jamil Ramji, Danielle Perry, Joey Ton, Nathan P. Beahm, Nicole Crisp, Beverly Dockrill, *et al.* "Simplified Guideline for Prescribing Medical Cannabinoids in Primary Care." *Canadian Family Physician* 64, no. 2 (February 1, 2018):111-120. cfp.ca/content/64/2/111.

Allan, G. Michael, Noah Ivers, and Charl Els. "Pharmacotherapy for Smoking." *Canadian Family Physician* 57, no. 1 (January 1, 2011): 47. cfp.ca/content/57/1/47.

American Cancer Society. "Cancer Facts & Figures 2003." Accessed February 27, 2018. whyquit.com/studies/2003_acs_cancer_facts.pdf.

American Cancer Society. "Health Risks of Smoking Tobacco." Accessed February 27, 2018. cancer.org/cancer/cancer-causes/tobacco-and-cancer/health-risks-of-smoking-tobacco.html.

American Cancer Society. "Quit Tobacco: How to Quit Smoking or Smokeless Tobacco." Accessed February 27, 2018. cancer.org/healthy/stay-away-from-tobacco/guide-quitting-smoking.html.

Benowitz, Neal L. "Pharmacology of Nicotine: Addiction, Smoking-Induced Disease, and Therapeutics." *Annual Review of Pharmacology and Toxicology* 49, no. 1 (2009): 57-71. doi:10.1146/annurev.pharmtox.48.113006.094742.

Benowitz, Neal L., Janne Hukkanen, and Peyton Jacob. "Nicotine Chemistry, Metabolism, Kinetics and Biomarkers." *Handbook of Experimental*

Pharmacology Nicotine Psychopharmacology 192 (2009): 29-60. doi:10. 1007/978-3-540-69248-5_2.

Cahill Kate, Nicola Lindson-Hawley, Kyla H. Thomas, Thomas R. Fanshawe, Tim Lancaster. "Nicotine Receptor Partial Agonists for Smoking Cessation." *Cochrane Database of Systematic Reviews* 5 (May 9 2016). doi:10.1002/14651858.CD006103.pub7.

Carr, Allen. *The Easy Way to Stop Smoking.* New York: Sterling, 2010.

Centre for Addiction and Mental Health. "Mental Illness & Addiction Index." Accessed February 27, 2018. camh.ca/en/health-info/ mental-illness-and-addiction-index.

Chaiton Michael, Lori Diemert, Joanna E. Cohen, Susan J. Bondy, Peter Selby, Anne Philipneri, and Robert Schwartz. "Estimating the Number of Quit Attempts It Takes to Quit Smoking Successfully in a Longitudinal Cohort of Smokers." *BMJ Open* 6, no. 6 (2016). doi:10.1136/bmjopen-2016-011045.

Evans, Dr. Mike. "What Is the Single Best Thing You Can Do to Quit Smoking?" DocMikeEvans, December 12, 2012. Video, 12:47. youtube.com/ watch?v=z16vhtjWKLO.

Gavura, Scott. "Medical Marijuana: Where Is the Evidence?" *Science-Based Medicine*, January 12, 2018, sciencebasedmedicine.org/medical-marijuana-where-is-the-evidence/.

Heath, Chip, and Dan Heath. *Switch: How to Change Things When Change Is Hard.* New York: Random House, 2013.

National Institutes of Health. "Reasons to Quit." Smokefree.gov. Accessed February 27, 2018. smokefree.gov/quitting-smoking/reasons-quit.

Stead, Lindsay F., Rafael Perera, Chris Bullen, David Mant, Jamie Hartmann-Boyce, Kate Cahill, and Tim Lancaster. "Nicotine Replacement Therapy for Smoking Cessation." *Cochrane Database of Systematic Reviews* 11 (2012). doi:10.1002/14651858.CD000146.pub4.

Chapter 8: Vaccinate

American Lung Association. "Trends in Pneumonia and Influenza Morbidity and Mortality." Epidemiology and Statistics Unit, Research and Health Education Division. November 2015. lung.org/assets/documents/research/ pi-trend-report/pdf.

Berkovic, Samuel F., Louise Harkin, Jacinta M. McMahon, James T. Pelekanos, Sameer M. Zuberi, Elaine C. Wirrell, Deepak S. Gill, Xenia Iona, John C. Mulley, and Ingrid E. Scheffer. "De-novo Mutations of the Sodium Channel Gene *SCN1A* in Alleged Vaccine Encephalopathy: A Retrospective Study." *The Lancet Neurology* 5, no. 6 (June 2006): 488-492. doi:10.1016/ s1474-4422(06)70446-x.

Bernard, Sallie. Comment on "Association Between Thimerosal-Containing Vaccine and Autism." *Jama* 291, no. 2 (2004): 180. doi:10.1001/ jama.291.2.180-b.

Caulfield, Timothy A., and Cindy Baker. *The Vaccination Picture.* Toronto: Penguin Canada, 2017.

Centers for Disease Control and Prevention. "Estimating Seasonal Influenza-Associated Deaths in the United States." National Center for Immunization and Respiratory Diseases. Updated January 29, 2018. cdc.gov/flu/about/ disease/us_flu-related_deaths.htm.

Centers for Disease Control and Prevention. "Immunization." National Center for Health Statistics. Updated May 3, 2017. cdc.gov/nchs/fastats/immunize. htm.

Centers for Disease Control and Prevention. "Seasonal Influenza-Associated Hospitalizations in the United States." National Center for Immunization and Respiratory Diseases. Updated December 9, 2016. cdc.gov/flu/about/ qa/hospital.htm.

Centers for Disease Control and Prevention. "Selected Publications on Influenza Vaccine Effectiveness." National Center for Immunization and Respiratory Diseases. Updated September 19, 2014. cdc.gov/flu/about/qa/ publications.htm.

Cherry, James D., Philip A. Brunell, Gerald S. Golden, and David T. Karzon. "Report of the Task Force on Pertussis and Pertussis Immunization—1988." *Pediatrics* 81, no. 6 (June 1988): 933-984.

DeStefano, Frank, and Robert T. Chen. "Negative Association between MMR and Autism." *The Lancet* 353, no. 9169 (June 12, 1999): 1987-1988. doi:10.1016/s0140-6736(99)00160-9.

Gorney, Cynthia. "Here's Why Vaccines Are So Crucial." *National Geographic*, November 2017, nationalgeographic.com/magazine/2017/11/ vaccine-health-infection-global-children/.

Haelle, Tara, and Emily Jane Willingham. "Vaccines: One Has an Evidence Base." In *The Informed Parent: A Science-Based Resource for Your Child's First Four Years*, 93-117. New York: Penguin Group, 2016.

Haelle, Tara. "Setting the Record Straight: Debunking ALL the Flu Vaccine Myths." *Red Wine & Apple Sauce*, October 28, 2013, redwineandapplesauce. com/2013/10/28/setting-the-record-straight-dubunking-all-the-flu-vaccine-myths/.

Majumder, Maimuna S., Emily L. Cohn, Sumiko R. Mekaru, Jane E. Huston, and John S. Brownstein. "Substandard Vaccination Compliance and the 2015 Measles Outbreak." *JAMA Pediatrics* 169, no. 5 (2015): 494. doi:10.1001/jamapediatrics.2015.0384.

Miller, D.L., E.M. Ross, R. Alderslade, M.H. Bellman, and N.S. Rawson. "Pertussis Immunisation and Serious Acute Neurological Illness in Children." *British Medical Journal* 282, no. 6279 (1981): 1595-1599.

Murphy, Trudy V., Paul M. Gargiullo, Mehran S. Massoudi, David B. Nelson, Aisha O. Jumaan, Catherine A. Okoro, Lynn R. Zanardi, *et.al.* "Intussusception among Infants Given an Oral Rotavirus Vaccine." *The New England Journal of Medicine* 344, no. 20 (February 22, 2001): 564-572. doi:10.1056/NEJM200102223440804.

National Vaccine Information Center. "Mercks's Gardasil Vaccine Not Proven Safe for Little Girls." Press release, June 27, 2006, nvic.org/nvic-archives/pressrelease/gardasilgirls.aspx.

Offit, Paul A. *Deadly Choices: How the Anti-Vaccine Movement Threatens Us All.* New York: Basic Books, 2015.

Offit, Paul A., and Charles J. Hackett. "Addressing Parents Concerns: Do Vaccines Cause Allergic or Autoimmune Diseases?" *Pediatrics* 111, no. 3 (March 1, 2003): 653-659. doi:10.1542/peds.111.3.653.

Public Health Agency of Canada. *Vaccination Coverage in Canadian Children: Results from the 2013 Childhood National Immunization Coverage Survey (CNICS).* Ottawa: Public Health Agency of Canada, May 2016. publications.gc.ca/collections/collection_2016/aspc-phac/HP40-156-2016-eng.pdf.

Times Editorial Board. "Vaccination Rates Are Up in California, but Pockets of Resistance Still Threaten Everyone." *Los Angeles Times*, August 15, 2017, latimes.com/opinion/editorials/la-ed-vaccination-gaps-troubling-20170814-story.html.

Wakefield, AJ, S.H. Murch, A. Anthony, J. Linnell, D.M. Casson, M. Malik, M. Berelowitz, *et al.* "RETRACTED: Ileal-lymphoid-nodular Hyperplasia, Non-specific Colitis, and Pervasive Developmental Disorder in Children." *The Lancet* 351, no. 9103 (February 28, 1998): 637-641. doi:10.1016/s0140-6736(97)11096-0.

"WHO Warning as European Measles Rate Jumps from Record Low." BBC News, February 20, 2018, bbc.com/news/health-43125242.

World Health Organization. "Immunization Coverage." Updated April 11, 2018. who.int/mediacentre/factsheets/fs378/en/.

World Health Organization. "Poliomyelitis Global Annual Reported Cases and Pol3 Coverage, 1980-2016." Updated August 2, 2017. who.int/immunization/monitoring_surveillance/burden/vpd/surveillance_type/active/Polio_coverage.jpg?ua+1.

World Health Organization. *2017 Assessment Report of the Global Vaccine Action Plan Strategic Advisory Group of Experts on Immunization.* Geneva: World Health Organization, 2017.

Chapter 9: Screen

Allan, G. Michael, Adrienne J. Lindblad, Ann Comeau, John Coppola, Brianne Hudson, Marco Mannarino, Cindy McMinis, *et al.* "Simplified Lipid Guidelines." *Canadian Family Physicians* 61, no. 10 (October 1, 2015): 857–867. cfp.ca/content/61/10/857.

American Society of Clinical Oncology. "Bladder Cancer: Statistics." Cancer.net. Updated October 2017. cancer.net/cancer-types/bladder-cancer/statistics.

Canadian Task Force on Preventive Health Care. "Abdominal Aortic Aneurysm (2017)." Accessed February 28, 2018. canadiantaskforce.ca/ guidelines/published-guidelines/abdominal-aortic-aneurysm/.

Canadian Task Force on Preventive Health Care. "Abdominal Aortic Aneurysm (AAA)-1000-Person Tool." Accessed February 28, 2018. canadiantaskforce. ca/tools-resources/abdominal-aortic-aneurysm-harms-and-benefits/.

Canadian Task Force on Preventive Health Care. "Breast Cancer—Risks & Benefits, Age 40–49." Accessed February 28, 2018. canadiantaskforce.ca/ tools-resources/breast-cancer-2/breast-cancer-risks-benefits-age-40-49/.

Canadian Task Force on Preventive Health Care. "Breast Cancer—Risks & Benefits, Age 50–69." Accessed February 28, 2018. canadiantaskforce.ca/ tools-resources/breast-cancer-2/breast-cancer-risks-benefits-age-50-69/.

Canadian Task Force on Preventive Health Care. "Cervical Cancer (2013)." Accessed February 28, 2018. canadiantaskforce.ca/guidelines/ published-guidelines/cervical-cancer/.

Canadian Task Force on Preventive Health Care. "Colorectal Cancer (2016)." Accessed February 28, 2018. canadiantaskforce.ca/guidelines/ published-guidelines/colorectal-cancer/.

Canadian Task Force on Preventive Health Care. "Diabetes, Type 2 (2012)." Accessed February 28, 2018. canadiantaskforce.ca/guidelines/ published-guidelines/type-2-diabetes/.

Canadian Task Force on Preventive Health Care. "Hypertension (2012)." Accessed February 28, 2018. canadiantaskforce.ca/guidelines/ published-guidelines/hypertension/.

Canadian Task Force on Preventive Health Care. "Lung Cancer (2016)." Accessed February 28, 2018. canadiantaskforce.ca/guidelines/ published-guidelines/lung-cancer/.

Canadian Task Force on Preventive Health Care. "Pelvic Exam (2016)." Accessed February 28, 2018. canadiantaskforce.ca/guidelines/ published-guidelines/pelvic-exam/.

Canadian Task Force on Preventive Health Care. "Prostate Cancer (2014)." Accessed February 28, 2018. canadiantaskforce.ca/guidelines/ published-guidelines/prostate-cancer/.

Canadian Task Force on Preventive Health Care. "Prostate Cancer-1000-Person Tool." Accessed February 28, 2018. canadiantaskforce.ca/tools-resources/prostate-cancer-harms-and-benefits/.

Canadian Task Force on Preventive Health Care. "Published Guidelines." Accessed February 28, 2018. canadiantaskforce.ca/guidelines/published-guidelines.

Hypertension Canada. "Goals of Therapy for Adults with Hypertension Without Compelling Indications for Specific Agents." From *Hypertension Canada's 2018 Guidelines for Diagnosis, Risk Assessment, Prevention, and Treatment of Hypertension in Adults and Children*. Accessed February 28, 2018. guidelines.hypertension.ca/prevention-treatment/uncomplicated-hypertension-goals-of-therapy/.

National Institute for Public Health and the Environment. "Cervical Cancer Screening in the Netherlands." RIVM. Updated October 20, 2016. rivm.nl/en/Documents_and_publications/Common_and_Present/Newsmessages/2014/Cervical_cancer_screening_in_the_Netherlands.

Papaioannou, Alexandra, Suzanne Morin, Angela M. Cheung, Stephanie Atkinson, Jacques P. Brown, Sidney Feldman, David A. Hanley, *et al.* "2010 Clinical Practice Guidelines for the Diagnosis and Management of Osteoporosis in Canada: Summary." *Canadian Medical Association Journal* 182, no. 17 (2010): 1864-1873. doi:10.1503/cmaj.100771.

US Preventive Services Task Force. *Final Update Summary: Abdominal Aortic Aneurysm: Screening*. June 2014. uspreventiveservicestaskforce.org/Page/Document/UpdateSummaryFinal/abdominal-aortic-aneurysm-screening.

US Preventive Services Task Force. *Final Update Summary: Abnormal Blood Glucose and Type 2 Diabetes Mellitus: Screening*. October 2015. uspreventiveservicestaskforce.org/Page/Document/UpdateSummaryFinal/screening-for-abnormal-blood-glucose-and-type-2-diabetes.

US Preventive Services Task Force. *Final Update Summary: Breast Cancer: Screening*. February 2018. uspreventiveservicestaskforce.org/Page/Document/UpdateSummaryFinal/breast-cancer-screening1?ds=1&s=breast.

US Preventive Services Task Force. *Final Update Summary: Cervical Cancer: Screening*. March 2012. uspreventiveservicestaskforce.org/Page/Document/UpdateSummaryFinal/cervical-cancer-screening.

US Preventive Services Task Force. *Final Update Summary: Colorectal Cancer: Screening*. June 2016. uspreventiveservicestaskforce.org/Page/Document/UpdateSummaryFinal/colorectal-cancer-screening2.

US Preventive Services Task Force. *Final Update Summary: Lung Cancer:*

Screening. December 2013. uspreventiveservicestaskforce.org/Page/
Document/UpdateSummaryFinal/lung-cancer-screening.

US Preventive Services Task Force. *Final Update Summary: Osteoporosis:
Screening.* January 2011. uspreventiveservicestaskforce.org/Page/
Document/UpdateSummaryFinal/osteoporosis-screening.

US Preventive Services Task Force. *Final Update Summary: Prostate Cancer:
Screening.* May 2012. uspreventiveservicestaskforce.org/Page/Document/
UpdateSummaryFinal/prostate-cancer-screening.

US Preventive Services Task Force. "USPSTF A and B Recommendations."
March 2018. uspreventiveservicestaskforce.org/Page/Name/
uspstf-a-and-b-recommendations.

Welch, H. Gilbert. *Should I Be Tested for Cancer?: Maybe Not and Here's Why.*
Berkeley, CA: University of California Press, 2006.

Woloshin, Steven, Lisa M. Schwartz, and H. Gilbert Welch. "Risk Charts:
Putting Cancer in Context." *Journal of the National Cancer Institute* 94, no.
11 (2002): 799–804. doi:10.1093/jnci/94.11.799.

Chapter 10: Supplement?

Allan, G. Michael, and Alma Bencivenga. "Vitamin D and Low Mood:
The Easy Perky Pill." Tools for Practice, Alberta College of Family
Physicians, June 23, 2014. acfp.ca/wp-content/uploads/tools-for-pract
ice/1404510453_20140623_093718.pdf.

Allan, G. Michael, and Frank Martino. "Vitamin D and Respiratory
Tract Infections: Does the Sun's Vitamin Chase the Cold?" Tools
for Practice, Alberta College of Family Physicians, October 27,
2014. acfp.ca/wp-content/uploads/tools-for-practice/1416503637_
tfpvitdandurtifvupdated.pdf.

Bjelakovic, Goran, Lise Lotte Gluud, Dimitrinka Nikolova, Kate Whitfield,
Jorn Wetterslev, Rosa G. Simonetti, Marija Bjelakovic, and Christian
Gluud. "Vitamin D Supplementation for Prevention of Mortality in
Adults." *Cochrane Database of Systematic Reviews* 1 (January 10, 2014).
doi:10.1002/14651858.CD007470.pub3.

Crislip, Mark. "Probiotics," *Science-Based Medicine*, February 10, 2017,
sciencebasedmedicine.org/probiotics/.

Ernst, Edzard. "Acupuncture—A Critical Analysis." *Journal
of Internal Medicine* 259, no. 2 (February 2006): 125–137.
doi:10.1111/j.1365-2796.2005.01584.x.

Ernst, Edzard, and Peter H. Canter. "A Systematic Review of Systematic
Reviews of Spinal Manipulation." *Journal of the Royal Society of Medicine* 99,
no. 4 (April 2006): 192–196. doi:10.1177/014107680609900418.

Gavura, Scott. "New Concerns about the Safety and Quality of Herbal Supplements." *Science-Based Medicine*, March 20, 2017, sciencebasedmedicine. org/new-concerns-about-the-safety-and-quality-of-herbal-supplements/.

Gavura, Scott. "Searching for the Supplement in Your Supplement." *Science-Based Medicine*, December 30, 2016, sciencebasedmedicine.org/ searching-for-the-supplement-in-your-supplement/.

Gavura, Scott. "What's in Your Supplement?" *Science-Based Medicine*, April 14, 2017, sciencebasedmedicine.org/whats-in-your-supplement/.

Gorski, David. "Alternative Medicine Kills Cancer Patients." *Science-Based Medicine*, November 24, 2017, sciencebasedmedicine.org/ alternative-medicine-kills-cancer-patients/.

Grant, Meghan. "Parents' Convictions in Son's Meningitis Death Upheld by Alberta Appeal Court." CBC News, November 16, 2017, cbc.ca/news/ canada/calgary/david-collet-stephan-meningitis-death-son-failure-provide-necessaries-appeal-1.4402665.

Davidson, Jonathan, Kishore M. Gadde, John Fairbank, K. Ranga Rama Krishnan, Robert M. Califf, Cynthia Binanay, Corette B. Parker, *et al.* "Effect of Hypericum perforatum (St John's Wort) in Major Depressive Disorder." *Jama* 287, no. 14 (April 2002): 1807. doi:10.1001/jama.287.14.1807.

Han, Esther, Nathalie Johnson, Tammy Delamelena, Margaret Glissmeyer, and Kari Steinbock. "Alternative Therapy Used as Primary Treatment for Breast Cancer Negatively Impacts Outcomes." *Annals of Surgical Oncology* 18, no. 4 (2011): 912-916. doi:10.1245/s10434-010-1487-0.

Hemilä, Harri, and Elizabeth Chalker. "Vitamin C for Preventing and Treating the Common Cold." *Cochrane Database of Systematic Reviews* 1 (January 31, 2013). doi:10.1002/14651858.CD000980.pub4.

Homola, Sam. "Neck Manipulation, Stroke, and the Vertebral Artery Stretch: Views, Opinions, and Options." *Science-Based Medicine*, September 1, 2017, sciencebasedmedicine.org/neck-manipulation-stroke-and-the-vertebral-artery-stretch-views-opinions-and-options/.

HOPE and HOPE-TOO Trial Investigators. "Effects of Long-term Vitamin E Supplementation on Cardiovascular Events and Cancer." *Jama* 293, no. 11 (2005): 1338-1347. doi:10.1001/jama.293.11.1338.

Labos, Christopher. "The Hard-to-Swallow Truth about Vitamin Pills." Macleans.ca. June 21, 2015. macleans.ca/society/health/ the-hard-to-swallow-truth-about-vitamin-pills/.

National Center for Complementary and Integrative Health. "Echinacea." Updated September 2016. nccih.nih.gov/health/echinacea/ataglance.htm.

National Institutes of Health. "Multivitamin/mineral Supplements." NIH

Office of Dietary Supplements. Updated July 8, 2015. ods.od.nih.gov/
factsheets/MVMS-HealthProfessional/.

National Institutes of Health. "Saw Palmetto." National Center for
Complementary and Integrative Health. Updated December 1, 2016. nccih.
nih.gov/health/palmetto/ataglance.htm.

Novella, Steven. "Herbal Medicine and Aristolochic Acid Nephropathy."
Science-Based Medicine, April 11, 2012, sciencebasedmedicine.org/
herbal-medicine-and-aristolochic-acid-nephropathy/.

Offit, Paul A. *Do You Believe in Magic?: Vitamins, Supplements, and All Things
Natural: A Look Behind the Curtain*. New York: HarperCollins, 2014.

Puckett, Renee M., and Martin Offringa. "Prophylactic Vitamin K for Vitamin
K Deficiency Bleeding in Neonates." *Cochrane Database of Systematic
Reviews* 4 (October 23, 2000). doi:10.1002/14651858.CD002776.

Rosa, Linda, Emily Rosa, Larry Sarner, and Stephen Barrett. "A Close Look at
Therapeutic Touch." *Jama* 279, no. 13 (April 1, 1998): 1005. doi:10.1001/
jama.279.13.1005–1010.

Rubinstein, S.M., M. van Middelkoop, W J. Assendelft, M.R. de Boer, and
M.W. van Tulder. "Spinal Manipulative Therapy for Chronic Low-Back
Pain." *Cochrane Database of Systematic Reviews* 2 (February 16, 2011).
doi:10.1002/14651858.CD008112.pub2.

Schwenger, Erin M., Aaron J. Tejani, and Peter S. Loewen. "Probiotics
for Preventing Urinary Tract Infections in Adults and Children."
Cochrane Database of Systematic Reviews 12 (December 23, 2015).
doi:10.1002/14651858.CD008772.pub2.

Singh, Simon, and E. Ernst. *Trick or Treatment: Alternative Medicine on Trial*.
London: Transworld, 2009.

Sulli, Maria Marzella, and Danielle C. Ezzo. "Drug Interactions with Vitamins
and Minerals." *U.S. Pharmacist*, January 23, 2007, uspharmacist.com/
article/drug-interactions-with-vitamins-and-minerals.

Tacklind, James, Roderick MacDonald, Indy Rutks, Judith U. Stanke, and
Timothy J. Wilt. "*Serenoa repens* for Benign Prostatic Hyperplasia."
Cochrane Database of Systematic Reviews 12 (December 12, 2012).
doi:10.1002/14651858.CD001423.pub3.

Tomassoni, Anthony J., and Karen Simone. "Herbal Medicines for Children:
An Illusion of Safety?" *Current Opinion in Pediatrics* 13, no. 2 (May 2001):
162–169. doi:10.1097/00008480-200104000-00014.

Weil, Andrew, and Brian Becker. "Dr. Weil's Personal Vitamin Routine."
DrWeil.com. Updated March 4, 2014. drweil.com/health-wellness/
balanced-living/meet-dr-weil/dr-weils-personal-vitamin-routine/.

White, Peter, Felicity L. Bishop, Phil Prescott, Clare Scott, Paul Little, and George Lewith. "Practice, Practitioner, or Placebo? A Multifactorial, Mixed-methods Randomized Controlled Trial of Acupuncture." *Pain* 153, no. 2 (February 2012): 455–462. doi:10.1016/j.pain.2011.11.007.

Acknowledgments

I HAD KEPT THE project of writing this book pretty close to the vest and only started talking about it openly as it neared completion. Despite that, there are a number of people who have helped me to stay inspired and motivated to keep on writing. First, I would like to thank all the people who are doing so much incredible work in promoting quality lifestyle advice and quelling the rise of pseudoscience—your work prompted me to join in and add one more voice to this important effort. Here are some writers, physicians, and speakers I would like to acknowledge: Mike Evans, James Fell, Yoni Freedhoff, Arya Sharma, Timothy Caulfield, Jennifer Gunter, Paul Offit, Simon Singh, Edzard Ernst, Michael Allan and James McCormack (*Best Science Medicine* podcast), Grant Ritchey Jr. and Clay Jones (*Prism* podcast), David Gorski, Steven Novella, Scott Gavura, Harriet Hall, and the rest of the team at ScienceBased-Medicine.org.

I need to also thank the team at Page Two Strategies for all their support and help in putting this together: Jesse Finkel-stein, publishing consultant, who believed in the project and helped me navigate the crazy and ever-changing world of publishing; Amanda Lewis, editorial director, who helped me turn something I felt reasonably happy with into something I can't wait to share; Crissy Calhoun, copyeditor, who cleaned up my writing even further and made me look like a better writer as a result; Gabrielle Narsted, publishing services manager, who always kept me on track with her efficiency and organization; Peter Cocking, creative director, who helped design a book with a look and feel I can truly be proud of; and Annemarie Tempelman-Kluit for her marketing expertise—an area in which I have needed much help.

There are a number of friends and family I would also like to acknowledge who inspired me to start writing this book, encouraged me to keep writing it, and/or provided help, support, and celebration at various points along the way: Trevor Langhan, Stephanie Tomilson, Vanessa Welch, Theo Versteegh, Julie Tripp, George Kim, Aaron Atcheson, Brad Turner, Darren Larsen, Angela Growse, Stephen Welch, Jeff and Laura Sandefer, my brother, Vinod Nair, and my parents, K.P.K and Radha Nair.

Finally, I need to thank my amazing wife, Andrea, for being the person who pushed me the most to stop talking about writing and to just do it. At an event, she announced to a group of friends that I was writing a book ... and so then I was. Andrea gave me the time to work on this undertaking despite how busy our family life already was. She has inspired me with her own writing ability and work ethic and helped immensely in the writing, editing, improvement, and promotion of this book. Andrea—and Kashi and Paxton—thank you for all your love, encouragement, and support. I couldn't have done this without you.

Index

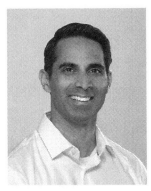

About the Author

DR. VINEET NAIR is a family physician and owner of the Core Family Health Centre, a multidisciplinary medical clinic. He has been passionate about primary care since he began practice in 2003 and has always been interested in the big-picture outlook on health and healthy lifestyles. In addition, Dr. Nair has been involved in primary care reform to find ways to improve the care that family doctors provide to patients, through the promotion of advanced-access scheduling, electronic medical record usage, and a focus on the fundamentals of healthy living. Dr. Nair is also passionate about education and is an adjunct professor at the Schulich School of Medicine & Dentistry at Western University. He is also the co-founder, with his wife, Andrea Nair, of Infinity School: An Acton Academy. They live in London, Ontario, with their two sons, Kashi and Paxton.

Learn more at:

CoreFamilyHealth.com

🐦 @VineetMD | 📷 @VineetMD | 📘 @VineetMD

MY GOAL IS for the *Healthier You* message to spread so that as many of us as possible can relax about the confusing information about health and focus our energy on what works!

To that end I'm continuing the *Healthier You* conversation online where you can get up-to-date information on my events and the resources mentioned in this book.

If you enjoyed *Healthier You,* and believe it's an important book that could help others improve their health, it would mean a lot to me if you'd take the time to leave a review on your favorite online bookstore:

* Amazon Canada
* Amazon US
* Barnes and Noble
* Indigo

If you would like to order more than 10 copies of *Healthier You,* please email **healthieryou@corefamilyhealth.com** and we'll get back to you with pricing and shipping details.

If you would like to promote healthy living at your home, office, or medical clinic, feel free to download the *Healthier You* poster from **www.corefamilyhealth.com/healthieryou** at no cost. Alternatively, if you would prefer having a bulk order delivered to you, please email **healthieryou@corefamily health.com** for further information on pricing and shipping.

Made in the USA
Middletown, DE
02 January 2020